Book De:

Whether you're a new parent or have done this before, you'll most likely be tracking every step along your baby's development, from their first smile to their first word. So many firsts to get excited about!

But one first that parents get a little freaked out about is potty-training. I know we all long for the day that we don't have to handle dirty diapers anymore, but the pressure of teaching our kiddies how to do something that should be so natural can be a scary prospect.

What if we teach them wrong? What if they don't get it? You may even have the dreaded thought that your girl will be the only child in history to get married wearing diapers.

Worries are normal! Potty-training is a step along the way to raising a happy, healthy child, and inevitably all parents worry about messing it up. On the other side of the coin, when we do start teaching, frustration can pop up easily.

Don't worry if you start to have thoughts like "Why can't she just figure out when she needs to wee?" Remember, even though it's a completely natural thing for us adults, we had to be taught too!

Your little girl is still a developing human. If we never taught her, she'd never know! It's up to us as parents to help guide our little ones in the right direction, and that's exactly what potty-training is.

Potty-training can be a worrisome and frustrating experience (for adults and children). But if you knew there was a way to get all the worry and frustration over with in just one weekend and come out of it with a potty-trained child, would you jump at the chance? I can't imagine many parents would say no to that!

This book is designed to be your guide to getting your daughter potty-trained in just three days. You'll learn how to:

- Identify signs that she's ready to start the process.
- Avoid mistakes that many parents make which drag the process out.
- Make the training stick.
- Deal with regression effectively.
- Have your daughter ready for big-world toilets using the 3-day method!

All you need is one long weekend of hard work, but it'll be worth it as you'll have your daughter potty-trained! Let's get started!

Potty-Training for Girls in 3 Days

A Step-by-Step Guide with Tips and Tricks for Modern Busy Parents to Potty-Train Their Toddlers

Stephany Hicks

© **Copyright 2020 - All rights reserved.**

The content contained within this book may not be reproduced, duplicated or transmitted without direct written permission from the author or the publisher.

Under no circumstances will any blame or legal responsibility be held against the publisher, or author, for any damages, reparation, or monetary loss due to the information contained within this book, either directly or indirectly.

<u>Legal Notice:</u>

This book is copyright protected. It is only for personal use. You cannot amend, distribute, sell, use, quote or paraphrase any part, or the content within this book, without the consent of the author or publisher.

<u>Disclaimer Notice:</u>

Please note the information contained within this document is for educational and entertainment purposes only. All effort has been executed to present accurate, up to date, reliable, complete information. No warranties of any kind are declared or implied. Readers acknowledge that the author is not engaged in the rendering of legal, financial, medical or professional advice. The content within this book has been derived from various sources. Please consult a licensed professional before attempting any techniques outlined in this book.

By reading this document, the reader agrees that under no circumstances is the author responsible for any losses, direct or indirect, that are incurred as a result of the use of the information contained within this document, including, but not limited to, errors, omissions, or inaccuracies.

Table of Contents

INTRODUCTION	**1**
THE PROBLEM	4
THE SOLUTION	6
About Stephany Hicks	7
CHAPTER 1: SETTING THE STAGE	**11**
HOW DO I KNOW MY DAUGHTER IS READY FOR TOILET TRAINING?	12
Signs to Look Out For	13
WHY CHOOSE THE 3-DAY METHOD?	17
WHAT IS REQUIRED TO USE THE 3-DAY METHOD?	19
The Right Frame of Mind	21
Potty Chair or Add-on Seat?	22
Big-Girl Panties	23
Treats and Rewards	23
The Right Diet	24
HOW WILL THIS BOOK HELP YOU?	25
CHAPTER 2: POTTY-TRAINING MYTHS AND MISTAKES	**27**
COMMON MYTHS	28
Asking Her If She Needs To Go	29
Your Little Girl Tells You She's Gone In Her Diaper, Now She's Ready to be Potty Trained	30
Rewards Are Necessary for Effective Toilet Training	31
Boys Are Easier to Potty-Train Than Girls	32
Your Daughter Will Tell You When She's Ready	33
Daycare Will Potty-Train Your Child	34
You Should Not Let Your Child Wear Diapers Once They Start Toilet Training	34
You Should Set Deadlines	35
COMMON MISTAKES	36
Rushing Your Daughter Into Potty-Training	36
Choosing the Wrong Time to Start	36
Having Unrealistic Expectations	37
Getting Upset About Accidents	37
Sticking With a Method That's Not Working	38
Forgetting How Your Child Is Feeling	39
Worrying That You're Doing It Wrong	39
Comparing Yourself/Your Child to Others	40
CHAPTER 3: PREPARATION	**43**

PREPARING YOUR DAUGHTER	44
Start Educating Her	45
Let Her Observe	45
Encourage Curiosity	46
Get Her Excited About It	47
PARENTAL PREPARATION	48
Schedule the Weekend	48
Get the Other Kids Out for the Weekend	49
Cheerleading and Tracking Success	50
Stock Up on Supplies	51
Meals	51
Snacks	52
Cleaning Supplies	53
CHAPTER 4: DAY 1	**55**
STEP 1 - FIRST YOU NEED TO START YOUR DAY	57
STEP 2 - GET HER EXCITED ABOUT IT	58
STEP 3 - EXPLAIN THE BASICS	59
STEP 4 - BE ATTENTIVE	60
THINGS TO REMEMBER	61
Accidents Are Going to Happen	61
Praise Her When She Does It Right	62
Be Careful How You Say Things	63
Make Sure Your Daughter Is Ready Before Beginning	63
CHAPTER 5: DAYS TWO AND THREE	**67**
STEPS TO FOLLOW THROUGH THE DAY	68
Keep Her Hydrated	68
Keep Her Eating	69
Keep an Eye on Her	69
Get Her to the Bathroom Quickly (When She Needs to Go)	70
Make Sure There Are No Distractions	71
THINGS TO KEEP IN MIND	72
Hand Washing	73
Wiping	73
Imitation	74
Positive Reinforcement	74
GETTING OUT OF THE HOUSE	75
Prepare	75
Be Quick	76
Be Calm	76

CHAPTER 6: AFTER THE THREE DAYS — 79

    REINFORCEMENT — 80
    DEALING WITH ACCIDENTS — 81
        What to Do in the Case of an Accident — 84
    REGRESSION — 85
        What to Do — 87
    COMMON PROBLEMS (AND THEIR SOLUTIONS) — 90
        Your Daughter Doesn't Recognize When She Needs to Go — 90
        She Resists Going to the Bathroom — 91
        She's Afraid of the Toilet — 92
        She Tries to Touch Her Pee or Poop — 93
        She'll Only Go to the Toilet With One Particular Person — 94

CONCLUSION — 97

REFERENCES — 101

Introduction

"Children are not things to be molded, but are people to be unfolded." - Jess Lair

I first came across this quote just after my daughter was born. I'd been given a lovely book as a gift, about having a daughter. It struck me, especially having two children already, that all the milestones we're so scared about as parents are simply our children becoming little people.

I was overjoyed to become a parent for the first time. Even the sleepless nights were a source of joy for me, and I relished every moment I spent with my baby. When it came to diaper changing, though, I was forced to hand over to dad or risk having to clean up more than just the poop.

When it came to potty-training, I was very happy at the prospect of not having to deal with diapers anymore. The poop would go where it belonged without dad or I having to get our hands on it.

It didn't quite go as I'd planned, though. I figured it would be simple - after all, it's a natural thing. Put baby on potty, let them do their thing, reward them, and next time it will go just the same way.

Well, it took a good many months before my first son got the toilet thing down. Those months were extremely frustrating. At every turn, I felt like I was failing my child! There were moments of tears from him, and moments of tears from me. I had irrational times when I worried that he would be stuck in diapers forever because of my failings as a parent.

Eventually, he did learn, but it was a much harder process than I expected. By the time son number two came along, I had some ideas of how to make the process easier. It still took a bit of time, but it took less time to potty-train my second son versus my first son.

A couple of years later, it was my daughter's turn. The panic flared up again, because you know, a girl is rather different than a boy. I had potty-training boys down to an acceptable art form now, but what about a girl?

Thankfully, I managed to reign in my fears and remain level-headed. I planned, I prepared, and I had an extreme determination to get this done in as little time and fuss as possible. And you know what? To my surprise, my preparation and plan worked. My daughter learned how to use the potty in just a weekend.

Yes! A weekend was all we needed to get her over this milestone. Of course, as with my other two, we had to deal with accidents, tears, fears, and worries, but we did it!

We went forward quite confidently, the accidents getting fewer and farther between until eventually, they stopped altogether. I won't lie - I was happy to have that part of parenting behind me.

It didn't take long, though, for me to realize that other moms I knew were struggling mightily with this milestone. My best friend and my sister-in-law both shared their potty-training struggles with me over the next few months. I witnessed their pains firsthand when accidents happened, and saw tears and frustrations from parents and children alike.

I was lucky enough to have some gems of information to share with these women, and I knew exactly how they were feeling at this point in their journey with their kids. Over wine and tissues, I shared tips and tricks that had worked with my three children, and gave some advice that I wished I'd had when I was going through the same things.

After discussing the pooping and peeing habits of our kids with a few of the women in my life, I had a light bulb moment. Every parent goes through this experience! I'd been lucky enough to have three runs at it, and I'd learned *a lot*.

I'd potty-trained boys. I'd potty-trained a girl. And with each subsequent child, it had become easier and quicker. In the space of two weeks, I'd heard from two struggling parents, and given advice that they'd taken and used.

I knew the hardships that came with potty-training, especially as both myself and my spouse were working. I can relate to the fear and irrational thoughts that can cross our minds when it comes to potty-training.

Why not share this information with more parents than just those close to me? Why not write all this advice down so that other struggling parents could be reassured, understand that they're not alone, and come to realize that there's an easier way?

With this in mind, I started to sit down and put my experiences on paper. I thought about what had worked well, as well as the differences between potty-training my daughter and my sons. I thought about the mistakes I had made along the way and if there was anything that had not worked. I realized that my daughter had learned a lot quicker than my two boys and I started to think about why. Before I knew it, I had gone through a whole writing pad and started to put a manual together that could help other parents.

This book is more comprehensive than the notes I had put together as I want it to add value. It's designed to be the foundation for potty-training, but with a specific focus on potty-training girls.

As you page through this book you'll find tips and advice as well as gain a better understanding for the following:

- Knowing when your little girl is ready to be potty-trained.
- We'll go through the myths and look at what's true.
- Go through the common mistakes and how to avoid them.
- Setting yourself and your daughter up for success.
- What to do if your child regresses.

- Turning lessons into potty-training habits that stick.

The 3-day potty-training method also allows you to customize the training to what you know would work best for your child. I can guarantee that the method, tips and advice in this book will work for 80% of children. You'll be able to use what works very well with your child, and adapt what you feel isn't working, so that you can successfully have your little one potty-trained.

By the time you've put this book down, you'll have a deeper understanding and a much better insight into potty-training. This will boost your confidence from the beginning and you won't have to wonder about your parenting skills. If you go through this confidently, your child will pick up on this, and she'll get through the training more confidently as well.

You may be wondering why this book is right for you? There are a number of potty-training books out there that you could choose from, so what makes this one different? For starters, the methodology found in this book works and it'll take less time for you to have your little girl potty-trained.

Why would you want to spend months, endless hours in the evenings after a long day at work, toilet training your daughter when you can do it in one long weekend? You may be thinking of sending her to a daycare, and she has to be potty-trained before she goes. The sooner you get her potty-trained the less stressed you'll be.

There will be moments when you find yourself thinking that potty-training is going to be like running a gauntlet. You'll find that it's not as difficult as you imagine it to be, I know as I've done it three times and it's a whole lot easier than you may think.

Why do some parents struggle with potty-training so much?

The Problem

As a little child, my father had a full-time job and my mother would stay home with us kids. My dad often left the house before we children were even awake, and mom would get us out of bed, make breakfast for us, and make sure we were entertained throughout the day while she cleaned the house. She'd make sure we were safe, well-fed, and got enough rest during the day, and still manage to make a hearty meal for my father. This way, all he had to do was sit down, and we'd start eating immediately when he arrived home.

Back then, there were no books and guides about potty-training your child. It was just something that all parents did, their own way. Although my mother didn't have guidelines on how to potty-train us effectively, she did have one thing on her side - **time**.

In between cooking us breakfast, cleaning the house, and cooking dinner, she had hours to spend with us kids. She had time and space to get creative when it came to teaching us how to use the toilet, and it was done over a period of time, because the time was there.

Today, though, many mothers work just as hard and long as dads do! Children spend less time with their parents and more time at daycare, and I can assure you your child is not likely to learn how to do the toilet thing at daycare. It's hard enough dealing with your own child's pooping habits, never mind teaching someone else's child how to use the toilet!

The fact is, many parents today simply don't have enough time to potty-train their children effectively (Bureau of Labor, 2020). Have you found this? Often, the first foray into potty-training goes something like this:

Saturday morning, we decide today is the day we're going to start teaching our child to use the big toilet. Saturday goes okay, and Sunday even better. Then comes Monday, and we're back to work but determined to keep it up. Monday evening we're a little tired, so we go to bed early, without really putting much effort into toilet training.

Tuesday is a bad day at work, so we just let our kiddie use the diaper without making mention of the toilet or potty. On Wednesday, we decide we'll pick it up again on the weekend, and so the cycle begins again.

When it comes to potty-training you need to be consistent from the start to finish. The only way to become good at something is through practice and working on it until we've nailed it.

One of the biggest and most common problems is working around schedules so that our kids can be toilet trained effectively.

The Solution

I know - if there was a parenting genie, most of us would wish to wake up tomorrow morning without kids already potty-trained. What if I could offer you the next best thing, though?

Imagine coming home on a Friday to a child wearing diapers and going to work on Tuesday with 90% of the potty-training done. All within one long weekend! Wouldn't you want to leap at the chance of your daughter being almost fully potty-trained in a weekend?

If it required some planning, some preparation, and a few weeks of laying the groundwork to give your child the best chance. Would you sacrifice three days so that your daughter can be potty-trained for once and for all?

Using the 3-day potty-training method is one of the best ways for working parents to potty-training their child effectively.

Just a weekend of hard work (after a few weeks of prep). There's no need to psych yourself up for months of wayward poop and wiping pee off the floor. Whether this is your first time potty-training or you've had to go through it before with your other child, the 3-day method is very effective.

It takes a bit of patience, following-up as time goes, and plenty of support and encouragement, your little one should be able to make the transition from being your little girl to being a big girl in just a weekend!

About Stephany Hicks

You may be asking who Stephany Hicks is. I'm a proud mom of three children, 2 sons and a daughter and all three are in college now.

That means I've been through the potty-training milestone three times! It was quite apparent to me that each one of my children responded quite differently to being potty-trained, so I spent a whole lot of time researching and putting into practice as many tips and tricks as I could find.

As well as potty-training my own children effectively, I've been lucky enough to have been able to give many of my own friends and family advice on how to potty-train their own children quickly and easily. When you've been through the same thing three times with different kiddies, different methods, but the same results, you come out with a good understanding of the troubles, fears and the feelings, troubles that come with it!

Helping you get through this process with minimal stress is important to me. It took me a trio of tries to figure out what works and what really doesn't, and to find a process that's both effective and fairly stress-free, for both the big and the little people involved.

Parents, I know how brutal this process can be. I'm here to help. The stresses of potty-training can spill over into other areas of life. Nobody wants their kids' poop to be the reason for family fights or falling behind at work!

But I'm also very interested in making this process as easy as possible for your child too. Your kiddie is at an age where they're learning. They're extremely impressionable! Unnecessary stresses for your child can hamper their learning, and stresses for parents can lead to some toxic behavior. Part of the point of this book is to prevent things like punishing your child in front of other people, or embarrassing them without even realizing it.

Reaching this milestone shouldn't be such a big scary thing! I've written this book to let you know you aren't alone in this process. One of my biggest passions is helping parents to find the balance between their work and family life.

While it will require effort, time and some work, the great news is that it's easy and can be achieved by all. Let's get started with the quick potty-training journey!

Chapter 1:

Setting the Stage

Every child is different when it comes to potty-training, and just like other developmental milestones your kid isn't going to stick to a one-size-fits-all schedule. This might cause some concern for parents who have busy work schedules, as you may be wondering how you'll ever get your child potty-trained. Or you may be a bit anxious about when you may need to start potty-training your child. Having three children of my own, two boys and a girl, I understand the challenges that parents face and that each child will undoubtedly present their own challenges when it comes to potty-training. The best way to start the process of potty-training your child is by spending time with them as they'll start to indicate when they're getting ready for potty-training. You also understand your child and their needs, so if you have a shy child, then they'll be more comfortable with potty-training when you do it.

You also can't pay someone to potty-train your child for you or think that they'll be potty-trained in preschool. You need to help build your child's confidence, in a safe and comfortable environment for them, and they'll feel safer and comfortable at home with you. The good news is that you've got this book and you're readying and that's the first step to potty-training your little girl. You'll learn a few new things about your daughter and the training along the way. This will also be a fantastic time when you can bond even more closely with your child in a fun way.

You may feel pressure to make sure that your little one's potty-training is successful, but remember that you know your child best and you have been with her since the day she was born. You are the best person to figure out what will work for her and how to make it exciting so that your little girl will want to continue with the potty-training. There will be some speed bumps in the road to potty-training, but be patient and persevere. Sometimes all you need to do is make some small adjustments to get back on track.

The 3-day method is a foundation for you to build on. You'll find that the techniques are easy to implement, and they're very effective. Once you've had a look at the method you'll quickly adapt the methods to what will work well for your child. You'll be able to incorporate things that will keep your child's interest and as well as motivate them as you can tailor the training to your child, while keeping to the foundation of the training. Children learn very quickly when the topic is exciting, fun and engaging.

You may already be asking yourself if your little girl is ready to be toilet trained now or you may be unsure of what the signs are that your child is ready. In this chapter we'll look at signs your child may be showing that'll let you know that they're ready to begin. I'll also go through a brief outline of the 3-day method and how it works, as well as why you should use it over other potty-training methods. There'll be a checklist of the things that you'll need for the 3-day potty-training. This will help you to prepare in advance as well as prepare what your little girl would respond to. By the end of Chapter 1, you'll know if your little girl is ready and you'll be ready to go as well.

How Do I Know My Daughter Is Ready for Toilet Training?

You can expect your child to learn how to use the toilet between 18 months and 3 years of age, but you'll be able to tell when you're little one is ready for potty-training (Choby & George, 2008). There are also benefits of having your child potty-trained. There will be no more diaper changes and I can say that you won't miss those days, especially when you're having to handle poopy-diapers.

As you see your child's personality unfold, and they're exploring their surroundings more confidently, or they've become a bit more cheeky and opinionated, you may be tempted to start potty-training. But let's take a step back as this doesn't necessarily mean that your little princess is ready to move to the toilet. If you leap into potty-training your girl too early it can be frustrating for both of you and may have negative consequences later on. Don't compare your child's progress with that of your friends and families kids either. Every child marches to the beat of their own drum and even if you ask around, you'll find that everyone has a different answer. You're trying to master a fine line between ready to potty-train and not having your girl be in diapers for longer than she should be.

The good news is that your little girl will know when she's ready to be potty-trained and she'll show signs of this. You'll have to make sure that she's displaying two or more of the signs and that she's doing them more frequently. You may have even noticed that your child is staying drier for longer, which shows that she's able to control her bladder. Then you'll know that you'll be a little girl on her way to becoming a big girl.

Signs to Look Out For

Children often surprise us especially when they start to become more aware of themselves and their bodies. Their natural curiosity and their ability to learn about their own body and what they should be doing can happen very quickly. It's like something just "clicks" as they're exploring the world around them.

Your daughter will know when it's time to be free of the diaper although she may not understand or know that she needs to be potty-trained. She'll definitely show you signs that she's ready to put on the "big-girl" panties. As parents, we constantly have to remind ourselves that we can't force or rush the potty-training and to pay attention to the signs our little darling is giving us.

- **Showing Related Interests**

When your little girl starts showing an interest in the toilet, or what you're doing when you go to the toilet, the potty or in panties, then she could ready to start potty-training. She may ask questions about what you're doing and why or even why she is wearing diapers and not panties.

You may find that your little girl is showing more curiosity and will watch when you or her father go to the bathroom. She may also ask questions about why there's a difference and this will be the perfect opportunity to teach her the difference between boys and girls and why they use the toilet differently.

Children learn by imitating their parents, and one way you can help your daughter is by showing her how to sit on a potty by using one of her favorite dolls. This will help her feel more comfortable as well as see that there's nothing to fear from sitting on the potty.

If she has older siblings she may also watch and imitate them in the bathroom. You may have to explain to her that, while it's okay that she follows you and daddy into the bathroom, she can't follow everyone into the bathroom.

- **She's Becoming Uncomfortable**

Your daughter may be wiggling out of her diaper or tugging on it and saying that she's no longer comfortable in a diaper. Sometimes you can put a diaper on only to find that she's removed it and is running around wild and free. Don't be alarmed by this, it's perfectly natural although it can be a bit disconcerting if she does this while out at friends or in public places, especially if you don't know where the diaper is! There is a possibility of this happening.

She may become fussy when you're trying to put a diaper on her, and she complains that it's too hot or dirty. This could be a chance to introduce her to cool comfortable underwear that won't have her tugging at it. Be sure that she's showing discomfort at the diaper being full or saggy.

Your little girl needs to notice that she's no longer comfortable and that she's not picking up cues from you that you're not comfortable with the diaper. If she's been playing and the diaper is askew, this won't indicate that she's not comfortable with the diaper.

You'll have to be patient and try not to show any frustration when a diaper goes missing or when she fusses about you putting on another diaper.

- **She Expresses the Need to Go**

While she has gotten used to being able to go whenever and wherever she has been because of the diaper. Your little girl may become aware of what it feels like when she needs to go and is also becoming aware of bladder control.

She may start saying things like, "I need to go" or she may be showing it physically by crossing her legs or fidgeting. She may just go very quiet and may even move to another room or even under the table to relieve herself in her diaper. This is a sign that she's ready to be potty-trained as she's aware of what she's feeling.

Children may not always know how to say that they need to go, so it's important that you watch what her body language and what she's doing. Also be aware if they start trying to hide behind couches or under tables when they go in their diapers. This will allow you opportunities to introduce them to the potty in a healthy and exciting way.

- **She's Physically Able to**

Every child develops differently and just like some babies walk, run and balance at different ages the same can be said when it comes to potty-training. You want your child to be able to get on and off the potty comfortable and easily. Her coordination should be good enough for her to get on to the potty and hold herself upright while sitting on the potty. If she can't yet physically support herself, then she may not be ready for potty-training and you don't want to rush into potty-training either if she's unable to support herself.

You want your little girl to have as much independence as she can when she goes to the potty. This also goes for her being able to pull down her own panties and lift her skirt when she goes to use the potty. You don't want her becoming frustrated because she can't get to the potty because of her clothing.

You may also have to get her to practice sitting on the potty, even if she doesn't have to go. This will help her build her confidence in using the potty even if you're not around as she'll know exactly what to do.

- **She Is Imitating Others**

Kids learn by imitating either yourself, their dad or their siblings and this goes for potty-training as well. While they're imitating you when you're on the toilet, make it sound like it's fun and exciting. You can even get them to flush the toilet when you're done so that they can see that there's nothing to be scared of.

You can also take this opportunity to show them the "magic" of the toilet and how it makes things disappear. While she's imitating using the toilet, you can take this time to also get her familiar with good toilet hygiene, like how to use toilet paper and then washing her hands.

When you let her watch you, you're also helping her understand that it's normal and that everyone has to go to the toilet. You can even mention that it beats having a soggy diaper that keeps your bum wet all day. Also say, "Mum is having a wee" when you're on the toilet. All little ones love water and if you add a pink or cartoon character soap that she loves, she'll love to wash her hands too. This will get her into good hygiene habits.

You can even take these moments to teach her how to wipe properly as you want her to wipe from front to back. Getting her to wipe from front to back can be one of the more difficult challenges that you'll face, but also very important. As this can also help to prevent urine infections which can happen when girls start to potty-train.

- **She Has a Toilet Schedule**

Potty-training will be easier if your little girl has a toilet schedule in place. It can be difficult to keep track of unless she tells you before or just after you have put a diaper on her, that she has to go.

However, if you have kept to a diaper changing routine then your child may already be used to pooping or making a wee at the same time when the diaper has been changed. This is also a good sign that her body is developing well, that there is a degree of bladder control and that her body is doing what it should be. But this sign on its own shouldn't be taken as your daughter being ready to potty-train. There are a number of things to consider when looking at your little princesses toilet schedule, from fiber in her diet that could have her going to the toilet after lunch or it being warmer, and she's had more to drink than usual. You want to be sure that her body has created its own toilet schedule and that it's not because of what she has consumed.

If you're spending a lot of time with your kid and you stick to a strict meal and nap schedule then it would be easier to tell if she has developed a toilet routine. You'd also know what she's had to eat and drink throughout the day, and you'd know if it was something that her tummy was just processing or if it's more normal.

So if you've seen more than one of these signs consistently, then the chances are great that your little princess is ready for the next step. The only thing that is left is getting your daughter to use the potty consistently without giving a second thought to diapers again.

While everyone has their opinion on when and how this should happen, you know your little one the best. I know from my own potty-training experiences that things can go smoothly, there'll be bumps in the roads and before you know it, your girl is potty-trained. This is why I'm sharing the 3-day potty-training blueprint with you. You'll be able to tweak it to what best suits your kids needs.

Why Choose the 3-Day Method?

As much as we love our children, and as much as we love being parents, the one thing we can almost certainly agree on is that we don't look forward to changing diapers. There's nothing more that can leave you feeling a little deflated after a long day at work, being stuck in traffic and then coming home to change a smelly poop diaper. We all secretly dread changing diapers and can't wait for the day when our little ones are potty-trained.

Potty-training needs to be done and it doesn't have to be a long-winded and frustrating experience. I can guarantee that it can be done in three days with proper planning, patience and perseverance. Some people may roll their eyes at the mention of potty-training your girl in just three days. You may even see a few raised eyebrows or even have a snide remark or two. Just remember that no two children are alike and that kids respond to things differently.

What I can tell you is that you shouldn't let others' opinions, comments or advice put you off or make you feel like an inadequate parent. We all have our own way of doing things, this doesn't make them right or wrong. It means that there's more than one way of doing things that may or may not work with your little girl. From my own personal experience of having to potty-train my two boys and my daughter, I've used the 3-day method and it works!

This method worked so well for me that I'm passing it on to every parent I can, so that they can have the best potty-training experience. There's so much stress at work, with projects and deadlines that the last thing you want is the stress of having to potty-train for weeks on end.

This means that the potty-training won't interfere with schedules and you won't have to take time off from work. The world has become far too busy and often both parents have full-time jobs, this can make potty-training extremely difficult when time is limited. Between having to cook dinner, spend time with the kids, get them to bed, possibly do some more work at home, there's barely time left for you. The idea of having to potty-train your girl before bed, can be overwhelming. Using the 3-day training method you can do it over a long weekend or you can take one day off from work.

You'll still have to be patient with the 3-day potty-training method, but it'll be less frustrating than if you had to try and do it over a couple of weeks. Children are very sensitive to feelings, and they'll pick up if we're frustrated or annoyed. They might know what to do with the feeling or even understand why you're feeling that way. Your girl may even feel like they've done something wrong.

By getting the potty-training done in three days you're able to create an exciting environment that will encourage and offer positive reinforcement. This can help build up your little darlings confidence and self-esteem which is important. We can only help to shape our kids into positive beliefs about themselves until the age of seven. If they have negative experiences while potty-training that make her feel like she's always doing something wrong, it can have lasting effects on your child's self-esteem.

You also don't want to confuse your child by having them potty-train for an hour a day, then go spend the weekend at their grandparents where they get told how to potty-train differently. The staff at day care centers aren't there to teach your little girl how to potty train, however sometimes they may feel the need to take it upon themselves as they're seeing your child for a large portion of the day. All these different tips and methods that your daughter is exposed to could confuse her and set the potty-training back.

Once you've laid the foundation and potty-trained your girl in three days, you can tell your daughters grandparents and day care teachers what you've done so that they can get on the same page and help positively reinforce the potty-training.

What Is Required to Use the 3-Day Method?

There's a fair amount of preparation that's needed before you leap into potting training your little princess, but this will help you to achieve the best results over the three days. You won't have to go out of your way to prepare, but having a structured plan is always great as it helps to keep things on track.

You don't have to rush out and buy everything that you think you may need for the potty-training. What I've mentioned here is for a "basic potty-training kit," and there's still room for you to customize it to suit you, your family and your little one's needs.

It will help to follow it as closely as you possibly can and leaving one step or a tool out can lead to having less desirable outcomes. I like to use positive reinforcement like giving the child a healthy snack that they enjoy or a toy as they achieve milestones. How you would like to reward your child is entirely up to you and you can swap snacks and toys for something else that your child may be more responsive to, like a trip to the zoo or visiting a friend.

As we go through the method I'll give some more alternatives as we delve more into each step later on in the book. This will help you to achieve the best results over the weekend and get your little girl using the potty confidently.

Here is what you'll need to do to get great results.

Three Full Days With the Parents

You'll need to spend 3 full days with your child, so I don't recommend trying to start potty-training if you need to visit the grandparents or go out to another kids birthday party. This may be a little tricky if you have other children that need to be picked up or if they have sporting activities. If at all possible try and get their siblings out of the house; see if they can spend a weekend at a friends house or even at the grandparents if that's an option.

Get your spouse on board with the potty-training so that you both know what each other's role will be. If needed, prepare meals in advance that you can take out of the freezer and pop into the oven so that you don't need to spend any time cooking. Tell friends and your loved ones that you're not available for socializing that weekend.

Plan some fun activities for you and the little champion potty-trainer to be so that you can prevent any boredom. This can range from arts and crafts to baking cookies, if you like. This weekend has one goal...for your little girl to be potty-trained and make sure that there's commitment from everyone that will be involved. Every moment you spend with her can lead to an opportunity for potty-training and showing her how to get it right.

Taking three days to potty-training is a lot easier than trying to fit in an hour of potty-training every day for three or four months. You also don't want your little girl picking up bad habits from the other kids like wiping from back to front, which can lead to a urinary infection.

Your daughter is going to love spending so much time with you and you'll be able to keep her stimulated throughout the weekend. You can even create some toilet games that will reinforce the training.

The Right Frame of Mind

You know how it feels when you have to do something that you don't particularly enjoy doing. It can seem like it's going to take forever to get through that one task. When it comes to potty-training your child, you'll have to have a positive frame of mind and you'll have to remind yourself to be patient. We've all been here, we've all had to go through potty-training. It's just that we've forgotten how we must have felt when we first had to use the potty.

Your child will be watching you and your spouse, imitating you and taking cues from you. If you feel grumpy, annoyed or impatient, your little princess will pick up on it. Only she may think that it's because she's doing something wrong. Don't forget that children are very sensitive to others' emotions, but they don't always understand the reason for the emotion.

There will be speed bumps on this potty-training journey, but that's all they are. Your child will get the hang of potty-training especially if you make things fun and exciting. It will also help if she's relaxed and comfortable in her environment. Girls have an amazing ability to focus on one thing at a time at this age, and you can use that to your advantage.

As the weekend unfolds, be adaptable and, no matter what, be mindful of the following:

- Whatever happens, stay calm.
- Things happen, you can't rush potty-training, so be patient.
- Praise your child when she uses the potty.
- If you're feeling frustrated, look at what she's already accomplished.
- Remember to breathe, your girl will learn this at her own pace.

It's important that you're consistent with the potty-training and the rewards throughout the 3 days.

Potty Chair or Add-on Seat?

There are two types of potties that you can get if you don't already have one.

- A free-standing potty chair
- A kid-sized seat attachment for the big toilet

The free-standing potty chair is cute and it can be placed in the bathroom. This can give your daughter a sense of pride as she has her very own toilet that she can use. You can even get stickers so that she can decorate it and get excited about using it.

It's also the right height for a small child, and they'll find it easy to use. It will be far less intimidating than a big grown-up toilet. If your girl is a little bit scared of the big toilet then this will help them as they won't have the anxiety around using the adult toilet. While this doesn't have water in it, they can still have fun flushing the adult toilet once they've done their business and it's transferred to the big toilet.

The kiddie-sized seat attaches to the big toilet and it creates a comfortable seat for your toddler to sit on, just like mom and dad. This is a great tool for when you need to go and visit friends or family as you can pack it up and take it with you. There's no need for cleaning anything after your little one has done their business and the toilet has been flushed.

Depending on the height of your toilet you may need to have a little step in place so that your little girl can get onto it. You may need to see how your child feels about the adult toilet before putting this into place as she may be scared of falling into the toilet.

My one child preferred the free-standing potty chair in the beginning and after a couple of months graduated to using the toilet seat, once he was more comfortable. Either way, your daughter will feel like they're getting a new toy. You'll need to have one of the two before you start your potty-training weekend.

Big-Girl Panties

You've had a discussion with your little girl where you've told her that you're taking her to buy some "big-girl" panties. Get her excited about this and then let her choose what panties she wants. You'll need the panties before the weekend as well, so she can have a couple of days to build up excitement before she gets to wear them. See if you can get her as excited about wearing panties as she would be at the thought of her favorite princess coming to visit her.

You'd need to get about 20 to 30 pairs of panties. Accidents are going to happen, so she's always going to need spare panties packed into her backpack until she has full control of her bladder. The last thing you want is her to come home from daycare without panties. This also means that you won't have to do washing every day to make sure she has clean underwear to go out.

Treats and Rewards

These are meant to be used to reinforce the positive milestones achieved by your child as she's on her potty-training journey. Depending on what you feel comfortable with and what would motivate your little girl you can use the following:

- Prepare her favorite snacks
- Get some new toys, like a coloring book or small doll
- Create a progress chart with stickers as rewards
- Come up with "experience" rewards, like a trip to the zoo or visiting a friend

The progress chart with stickers can be used with mini-treats that could lead up to the experience reward. This way she can see where she is and what she still needs to achieve to get her reward. It will come down to what will work best to motivate your girl.

The Right Diet

You'll need to make sure that your princess has plenty of fibrous food and drink plenty of beverages, so that when the moment arrives they'll be able to use the potty. Your little girl will start to understand and recognize when she should go to the bathroom and use the potty. With all the beverages and high fiber food you'll be giving her, there should be plenty of opportunities.

You can create snacks out of the following:

- Apples
- Pears
- Banana
- Oranges

- Berries
- Coconut
- Avocado
- Grapes
- Melons

You can also create yummy ice-popsicles from coconut water and combine this with fruit; it should help move things along swiftly. Try and stay away from foods that would be more binding, like bread or brown rice, dairy products and processed food as these can make your little one constipated. Having a constipated daughter for potty-training isn't going to help. Start introducing the foods at least two days before the time so that the body can start digesting. This will make this work better.

Now that you've set the dates, have taken a day's leave, cleared your schedule, prepared everything that you need for the weekend including food and snacks. All you need to do is check one more time that you've got everything you need, and you're ready to begin the potty-training weekend.

How Will This Book Help You?

This book will provide step-by-step instructions to help guide you through the potty-training, as well as provide techniques and tips. This will help you to cater to your child's specific needs. You'll also have a better understanding of the challenges that many parents face when potty-training and how you can work around them to achieve the best results.

There won't be a need for sticky notes around the house or having to recall something from memory, as everything you need is right here in this book. There are also training myths and mistakes that we'll cover so that you can navigate your way through the potty-training. You'll be able to tackle your potty-training weekend with confidence and know that there's nothing to worry or be anxious about.

If you are comfortable and can have fun potty-training your little girl, then she'll have a wonderful experience, as well. This will make the entire process enjoyable and positive for all concerned. You may even get some funny snapshots for the family album or even some really cute video that you can show off in the years to come. She may not be thrilled about it then, but at least there will be some fond memories around going potty.

Chapter 2:

Potty-Training Myths and Mistakes

Potty-training can seem like you've set sail into uncharted waters, and this can leave parents anxious and confused about what to expect or what to do. This can lead to parents making mistakes unintentionally that can confuse the child and make the potty-training process more difficult. You may feel like everyone else knows what they're doing or that they're pro's because they make it look so easy. The truth is every parent has their own unique potty-training challenges that they face, because your child isn't like any other child.

Even if you're about to embark on potty-training your second child, you'll find that what worked the first time round, may have you pulling your hair out this time. I know what it feels like, I had to potty-trainthree children, and each one had their own challenges that I had to handle. You need to remind yourself that you know your daughter and that you know what she'll respond to. You can put the GPS coordinates into it and start sailing and everything starts off well, until your GPS needs to reroute, there're no landmarks to be seen and now you're not sure if you're heading in the right direction. It can be a scary place to be in, but if you trust your skills, your instincts and the knowledge that you have, you'll reach your destination, even if you take a detour!

All parents may take detours, but they reach the end destination which is a potty-trained little girl. There's no right way or wrong way and it also comes down to what you know your child will be comfortable with.

Google is not your friend when it comes to potty-training, as this can lead to information overload and leave you feeling dazed and confused. It's like trying to diagnose an illness on WebMD, you could have 10 different possible illnesses, but not a single match. There is some ridiculous information out there when it comes to potty-training, but I have found that training with positive reinforcement and encouragement has worked wonders.

To help you with this we'll discuss the potty-training myths, what happens to the body and why some of these things have become popular beliefs. There's no need for you to worry about them and once you've got the knowledge you'll have peace of mind on your own child's potty-training journey.

Let's have a look at some of the myths!

Common Myths

You should know that everyone is going to have their opinion on how you should potty-train your girl as well as give their advice. I know of friendships that have ended because discussions about potty-training have become that heated. Potty-training can be a very sensitive subject, especially when people are saying that a child should be potty-trained at 18 months or that you're taking the wrong approach. It can be difficult to listen to everyone's input. My advice is listen and take what would be good and see if you could use it in the 3-day training method.

This could be something other parents did that was positive and motivated the child to use the potty. At the end of the day, you know your child! If you decide to Google potty-training you'll come across some that have merit and some that will raise an eyebrow and some may even seem logical ... at first. It's good that you're looking for answers to help you on your child's potty-training journey and together we're going to give you some myths as well as why they're a little out there. This can be backed up by science, psychology as well as instinct and what we know about the human body.

We'll unravel the information for you so that you get to the truth of the matter, so that you can have a better understanding of what's false information, what's good information and what will give you, your child and your family a better potty-training experience.

I want to make sure that your child has the best experience when it comes to potty-training so that the lasting effects are positive. These positive effects will help your child with confidence and self-esteem in the long run. At the end of the day, you'll need to decide what will work best for your child, and if there's something that you see in this chapter, feel free to incorporate it into the 3-day potty-training. Just bear in mind that not everything works for every child and you need to keep your child in mind when going through the myths so you think about what may or may not work.

Let's get into the misconceptions of potting training!

Asking Her If She Needs To Go

Your little girl still needs to link the feeling of needing to go to the toilet with going to the toilet. Her whole life she's just gone in her diaper, and she's just starting to figure out bladder control and her diaper is staying dryer for longer. Now you're going to be asking her every 30 minutes if she needs to go to the toilet.

You want your child to be able to listen to her body and recognize that she needs to go to the toilet. Could you imagine if your manager at the office asked you every 30 minutes if you needed to go to the bathroom? Wouldn't that annoy you? Would you eventually get mad and tell her that you'll go when you need to?

Now, I know that may be ridiculous because a manager isn't going to ask you when you need to go to the bathroom. So why would you constantly ask your child if she needs to go when she's still figuring this out? If you were in your child's shoes, would you be somewhat confused if you're always being asked, "Do you need to go?" or "Do you need to poop?" Especially when you're still figuring this out. This will not build your child's confidence, and she may start to feel like there's something wrong with her. It can also lead to her feeling pressured. This can have a negative association with the toilet, which can make potty-training difficult. It may seem logical to ask your girl if they need to go to the toilet, but this doesn't stimulate the body to get the process going.

There's a link between the brain and the body that happens when someone needs to relieve themselves, and this link has to be developed (National Center for Biotechnology Information, 2019). You can't teach your daughter when she needs to wee, her body will tell her when she needs to wee, and this communication happens between the brain and the body. Do you remember what it felt like when you were learning to wee in the toilet and how you could tell if you needed to wee? Probably not. This happens naturally and without us having to give much thought to it.

You don't want your daughter to start thinking she needs to go and wee, especially when she's not feeling the need to go. This will leave her feeling frustrated and it can have a negative impact as she won't understand why she's not able to go when she thinks about it, as opposed to feeling it. Even more so, if they see how disappointed you are when you think the little one has taken a step forward and then nothing happens.

Your Little Girl Tells You She's Gone In Her Diaper, Now She's Ready to be Potty Trained

It's great when your little girl becomes aware of what is happening and that they need to be changed but this doesn't mean that they're ready to begin with potty-training. While she knows that her soggy diaper is uncomfortable it means that she's realizing the difference between dry and comfortable and wet and uncomfortable. While this can be a sign that she's ready to begin with her potty-training, you can't begin if this is the only sign. She needs to realize that she needs to recognize that when she needs to go and not that she has gone.

It's like driving to a new place, on a route that's unfamiliar to you. You'll follow the GPS but you may not realize that you've taken the wrong turn until it's happened. Thankfully, your GPS will correct you and get you to your destination. But there's a difference between knowing that you're lost and knowing a route or map well enough not to get lost in the first place.

If she wants to take her diaper off, or is telling you that she needs to be changed, then start looking for other signs that she's ready to be potty-trained. You want her to understand that she needs to tell you before she goes in the diaper and not afterwards. It's creating that link, so she can feel that she needs to go and then understand that she needs to go to the toilet.

There are a number of reasons why children complain about their diapers. For example:

- Their skin could be sensitive, and they don't like the feel of the cold, wet diaper
- You may have switched diaper brands, and she could find this to uncomfortable
- Labial adhesions and/or inflammation
- Urinary tract infection
- Yeast diaper rash

If your child doesn't have any of the above, and there are no other symptoms or signs, then give it some time before you start her on potty-training.

Rewards Are Necessary for Effective Toilet Training

Rewarding your little girl is helpful, but there are various ways in which you can reward her. Verbal praise can be just as effective as giving her a new toy or treat. We tend to show our affection by giving gifts to those we care about, and this is no different when it comes to our children. We want our children to have nice things and have the latest gadgets that can stimulate them, and we're all guilty of this, to some degree.

Your girl will respond to a hug, a high-five or any other means of encouragement as well. It helps to motivate your little girl when there's something that they really want, and they need to do well in order to get it. They also do need to be spoiled at times as well, but everything in moderation so that the child can grow up being well-rounded. They shouldn't expect a reward for doing something. There has to be a balance.

This doesn't mean that you shouldn't use rewarding techniques when it comes to potty-training. After all, you may reach for some candy and your little girl could refuse that reward and want a hug instead. If your child is terribly shy, then she may need an extra incentive for when she's battling with something.

You don't need to reward your child every time they use the potty, alternating with verbal reinforcement is just as effective when it comes to making the lessons effective and will stay with the child. At the end of the day, only you know your child and it's up to you how you choose to reward her. Some girls will learn quickly because they know that they ice-cream waiting for them. While other children may learn just as quickly because they're getting approval and verbal reinforcement from their parents. If you only have toys and treats lined up, the child could get bored with that and even become disinterested. You'll need to put some thought into what makes your child tick, and keep them interested.

When your little girl does use the potty, and gets the wiping from front to back, celebrate it! Lavish her with hugs, kisses and lots of love. Praise goes a long way and will usually do the trick for longer than toys or candy.

Boys Are Easier to Potty-Train Than Girls

I can't begin to recall how many times I have heard this. And as a mom of two boys and a girl, I can tell you that it isn't true. In fact, there's no evidence to support the claim that it's harder to potty-train girls than boys or vice versa. While the mechanics are different, and it's trickier for mom's to teach their boys how to do their thing, dad's may find it tricky to teach girls to do their thing. The hardest kids to train are the stubborn ones, and this can be a girl or a boy.

Every parent has their own experience with the child regardless of gender. After all, every child is different and each one will respond differently to potty-training. Children can be mischievous and sometimes they just don't want to learn how to be potty-trained. They can take it up a notch and behave like a brat. Whether it's a girl or a boy, they can both be little angels, which makes potty-training easier, or they can be stubborn, dig their heels in and refuse to be potty-trained. You know and understand your daughter and at the end of the day, you'll have to figure out what makes them tick to get the end-result of having them potty-trained.

Your Daughter Will Tell You When She's Ready

Your child is changing and developing all the time; they're exploring and learning new things and becoming more self-aware. This will continue for many years and it's part of their learning curve. When they're toddlers, they'll get distracted by different toys, noises outside and will go with the flow of what's going on. These are their carefree days, where they're discovering the world around them. Then they wake up one day and realize that girls and boys are different.

Their curious nature will have them asking a million questions and no answer will seem to satisfy this curiosity. But they're starting to notice that there are differences and that their bodies are different. Most of the time they don't know how to describe what they feel or what's happening, they just seem to take it all in their stride.

As your child learns how to use the toilet, they're not going to tell you that they're ready for potty-training. Your daughter doesn't quite understand her anatomy yet, or what the body parts are called, and she won't fully understand what she's feeling. As adults, we can be working behind our desk for hours. Suddenly, we feel a twinge near our bladder, and we know that we've had a lot of fluid, and we need to get to the toilet. Your little girl still has to learn and understand this.

If your spouse says, "Get ready - it's almost time to go," you know that you've got to touch up your lipstick, grab your coat, grab your comfortable shoes and leave. If you say, "Get ready" to your toddler, they may run outside to fetch the dog a stick or run to your bedroom and fetch your slippers as opposed to leaving the house. She doesn't know what that twinge in her bladder means yet, just like she's not going to go sprinting to the car when she hears the words "Get Ready." While your daughter may have an idea that the diaper needs to go, she won't know how to communicate this to you.

Daycare Will Potty-Train Your Child

There are a number of parents who assume that their child will be potty-trained by the daycare center staff, as they spend most time with your child during the day. But most day care centers require that your child is already potty-trained by the time that they're enrolled with the daycare center. Now let me ask you this, how would you feel about a staff member of the daycare center disciplining your child? How would you feel if that staff member smacked your child's hand when they did something that they considered to be inappropriate? Would you read them the riot act? Or would you take into consideration what your child did, and then decide if you're okay with the staff member disciplining your child?

Most parents are going to be upset if they heard that their child received a smack on the hand or the bottom, so why would you let a virtual stranger potty-trainyour child? It's an intimate lesson that your child needs to learn, and they should be in a comfortable environment where they're been shown how to use the toilet by someone that they trust. Potty-training can be valuable bonding time with your child that helps to further instill trust between the two of you.

You will be very lucky to find a daycare center who'll assist you with potty-training, however their method can leave your little one confused. Especially if you're also potty-training them in the evenings at home and over the weekend and asking them to do things differently. If you're not potty-training your child and leaving it up to the daycare center staff, you may have your child come home with some undesirable habits. You may find that the daycare center uses a toilet seat, while you're using the free-standing potty chair at home. This could cause some discomfort to your child and hinder the potty-training, as she may refuse to use the toilet seat potty.

You Should Not Let Your Child Wear Diapers Once They Start Toilet Training

It's a good idea to put a diaper on your little girl at night, as she's probably not going to wake up in the middle of the night to go to the bathroom. If she did, she may be afraid of the dark and won't leave the bed. It also wouldn't be a good idea to wake her up every 4 hours to go and use the toilet; you also need to be well rested for work.

The best thing to do is to use a diaper at night until you see that it's becoming dryer. You'd have to get your child into the habit of waking up and going straight to the bathroom to relieve herself.

She will eventually be able to control her bladder and not need to use a diaper. The diaper also helps to prevent her from wetting the bed, which can have a negative impact on her confidence and self-esteem. Your daughter may also see wetting the bed as her doing something wrong and can cause her anxiety in the evening.

Let her use the potty in the evening before you put the diaper on her, and she goes to bed. This will also help to see how wet or dry the diaper is in the morning.

You Should Set Deadlines

Setting deadlines is like setting yourself up for disappointment, and setting your girl up for failure. You can't predict when your daughter is going to have an accident or when they'll be fully potty-trained. You need to be patient and understand that these things can take time. You could also be putting pressure on your little one to potty train; this can actually hinder the potty-training as opposed to helping it along.

Every child is different, and the rate at which they become potty-trained is different as well. Some children can master the potty-training very quickly others will need a bit more work and reinforcement of the potty-training. Your child has a unique temperament, and she could very well be marching to a different development drum beat.

To see the best results, encourage, reinforce the potty-training and cater the potty-training to her individual personality. Make sure that the potty-training method that you use for your child is flexible and that she feels comfortable with it.

Common Mistakes

Potty-training is going to be one of the most difficult challenges that you're going to face. It would be marvelous if our little ones would potty-train themselves, but this is wishful thinking. As parents, we may feel like we need to get potty-training underway as soon as possible, but there are some common mistakes that parents make when it comes to potty-training.

Here are some common mistakes that parents have made.

Rushing Your Daughter Into Potty-Training

Potty-training is a developmental milestone for your little girl and you can't rush her into potty-training. You couldn't rush her into crawling, walking or even talking, so you won't be able to push them into potty-training before they're ready. If you do, your child can feel pressured, and she will simply withhold her poop. This will create a negative association, your little princess will become constipated and uncomfortable bowel movements. She won't want a repetition of this process, so she will begin to fight the urge to go and this only makes the constipation worse.

Your first instinct is to give her some pooping medicine, like a laxative, and then lure her back into the bathroom. But this can just make it worse and reinforce her fear of the experience. Before you jump the gun on potty-training, she must be able to control her bodily functions, and she also has to want to control her potty functions.

Before potty-training, make sure your little girl is showing more than one sign that she's ready to begin potty-training.

Choosing the Wrong Time to Start

When you're looking to start with potty-training, make sure that it's not going to be during a time when other life changing situations are occurring, like moving to a new house. You may want to put potty-training off if you're expecting another bundle of joy or if you're starting a new job. We often forget how sensitive our little ones are and how quickly they're able to pick on the emotions around them. If you're stressed or anxious about a situation then they'll be stressed and anxious but without knowing why.

Any new changes like moving to a new house can bring about excitement and worry of the unknown for your child. You don't want to be juggling new challenges and potty-training at the same time; this can lead to you feeling overwhelmed and frustrated. Plus, let's say your little girl isn't getting the potty-training method, and you have one moment where you shout at her out of frustration. This can make the whole potty-training experience a bad one for her, and it could take her a while to get over it.

Having Unrealistic Expectations

It's great if your friend Jenny's child is potty-trained and running around like a toilet warrior! Be happy for her and her daughter. Your little one has her own personality, and she'll be motivated by different things. When you're potty-training your princess, you can't have a time table, or deadlines so you're going to have to manage your expectations and make sure that they're realistic in terms of your little one.

There's nothing wrong if your child takes a bit longer or starts later than your friends' children, or your siblings' kids. Remember it's not a competition of whose little one was the first to be potty-trained or who got it the quickest. You need to go at your child's pace if you want potty-training to be successful.

Getting Upset About Accidents

Most of us had accidents as a child and you can expect your little girl to have a number of accidents. It's part of the learning process. The important thing to note is how you react to it. If your daughter has an accident while she's playing outside, don't say something like, "You're a big girl now, you shouldn't be having accidents" or "Why can't you get it right?" These will chip away at any confidence or self-esteem she has. Even worse, you'll reinforce the negative feeling she already has about the accident.

You want to reinforce that she can do it and that it may take some time. Tell her you love her and find a way that can make her feel better about going to the potty. I understand that it can be frustrating when your little girl has a number of accidents, and you feel like they should have "gotten it right" by now. Take a deep breath and think about the last time you had to learn something new and how you felt when you got things wrong. How would you have felt if somebody scolded you for doing something wrong when you're trying your best?

Our lives are busy, and we can feel tired most of the time. I understand that feeling too. But when it comes to a child who's still learning, you have to take a step back and be mindful that things don't always come naturally to all of us. Sometimes we need someone to be patient and be a cheerleader in our corner, even if there are mainly small victories that are celebrated. The small victories lead to the big ones.

Sticking With a Method That's Not Working

When you're baking, you want your cake to come out perfectly. It should be soft, fluffy and moist. Now if you're constantly getting cakes that flop from the same recipe, you're not going to stick with it. You'll find a different recipe and try that. It's the same with potty-training. Don't stick with a method if it's not working.

Both you and your little one are learning together as you follow the process. You'll need to be able to adapt and remain flexible so that you can incorporate different techniques, until you find the one that works with your girl. Baking a cake has the same ingredients to get the foundation of it; but if you want chocolate instead of vanilla, you'll add cocoa powder to it. Potty-training can be like baking your cake. There'll be some trial and error, but you can clean up the mess and try something different until you get your perfect cake, or in this case, your child potty-trained.

Forgetting How Your Child Is Feeling

I've said it numerous times through the book; our little ones are sensitive and, sometimes without realizing it, our actions can make our little girl feel pressured. She may even feel like she's doing something wrong, and she can sense that she's frustrating you. This can open up a can of worms that will lead to negative experiences and cause her to fear the experience entirely.

Be sure to chat with your girl and see how they're doing and if they're okay with everything. Bear in mind that they may not know how to express what they're feeling clearly. All you can really do is reassure them, tell them you love them, give them some hugs and move forward.

It's important that they have positive experiences throughout the potty-training, as this will help the training to stick. If you feel like your child may be feeling pressured, then it's okay to give the potty-training a break for a few days and then start again.

Worrying That You're Doing It Wrong

It's important for you to know that there's no right way or wrong way when it comes to potty-training. Children are different and they all learn differently. You can make potty-training fun and experiment with different techniques that can help your child grasp the potty-training. You know your child and you'll be able to find what works best for her, even if this means reading a book to her while she's on the potty.

There are going to be amazing potty-training moments and then there are going to be some low potty-training moments. This happens to all of us, and we all have to face the different challenges that our kids will throw our way. Trust your instincts as well; this can also help you to navigate what works and what doesn't.

Comparing Yourself/Your Child to Others

It can be difficult to see how your siblings or friends children have taken to potty-training, especially if they're seeing results. It can also be difficult to remind yourself that every child is different and that the developmental milestones are different, as well. You don't want to start comparing your daughter to other people's little one's since this can lead to immense frustration, for both you and your daughter.

It can also lead to you feeling like a bad parent and that you're doing something wrong. I can tell you, that you're not doing anything wrong and that you're not a bad parent! Every mom has a bag of ingenious tricks that she knows will work on her kids. Sometimes all you need to do is be a bit more creative and find what makes your daughter tick so that you can both enjoy the potty-training experience.

Chapter 3:

Preparation

If this is your first time potty-training, or you've already potty-trained a child, the one thing I can guarantee is that preparation is vital to the success of the potty-training. We plan for so many other things, like taking a road trip, moving to a new house or looking for a new job. This type of preparation helps reduce the stress of the process. It also allows for some flexibility if things change, like the moving truck arriving three hours late. This should be no different when you start with potty-training your daughter.

Preparation for potty-training has two sides that you must take into consideration:

- Preparation for the parents
- Preparation for your little girl

This will reduce the amount of anxiety and stress from potty-training over the three days as you know what you can expect. You already have an idea of what the common mistakes are, and you have a better understanding of the myths of potty-training. You also have this book, which will be with you every step of the way and this will help you manage your expectations as well as what you should be doing to have the best potty-training experience.

You and your spouse should have discussed the potty-training weekend, and both of you should be on the same page, and having had some time to think about what each one is going to be doing. Just remember, there's no good cop or bad cop when it comes to potty-training.

Your little princess, on the other hand, could be braiding the tail of her unicorn and getting it ready for the tea party that's going to be happening soon. She's probably blissfully unaware that she's going to be taking part in potty-training soon that will leave her diaper free and wearing big-girl panties. She may feel overwhelmed if it's sprung on her the day that you want to start the potty-training. While she may love surprises, potty-training isn't best left as a surprise.

You've gone through all the effort of making sure that she's ready for potty-training, which isn't easy, I know. It can be exhausting analyzing your little one's actions and behavior to see if they're ready for one of the biggest challenges they've yet to face. You've been watching her when she follows her dad to the bathroom to see what's going on. Maybe you've had to chase her through the house, her running wild and free with a diaper in her hand. All the while she's telling you that the diaper's dirty.

I know that it can be difficult to tell when you're little one is ready for the potty challenge and there's a part of us that wishes that she'd never grow up at all. We just want them to stay little and adorable forever. But, now that you're sure that she's ready to take the next development milestone step in her life, it's best to prepare her for what's to come over the long weekend.

Preparing Your Daughter

Congratulations on taking the first steps towards the big milestone of your daughter's life! The potty-training journey may have you and your spouse sitting on the couch Googling what the best potty is and you reading reviews to see what would be best. Your little princess is still unaware of what's to come. You and your spouse have decided on the best way forward for the potty-training. Now you just need to tell your little girl what's going to be happening.

When you start telling her that she's going to be doing potty-training, you want her to be excited about it. She'll more than likely bombard you with a million questions; she could resist the training from the start, or she may jump on board all excited. You can schedule the potty-training to happen two weeks from when you tell her, or for a month later. You'll know what works best for your little girl.

Get some child-friendly potty-training books so that she can have a better understanding of what's going to happen. If need be, get her magical unicorn involved since even the unicorn can join in the potty-training fun. You want her to feel that she's safe and that there's no pressure. Once you have her excited, there are ways that you can help get her involved in the process and get her ready for her potty-training "boot camp."

Start Educating Her

Potty-training is mastering the art of where to go when your little girl needs to go. This is the important factor that she will have to understand. So far, for her whole life, she's been able to go exactly where she has been standing, sitting or playing. While having a wee or a poo is a natural bodily function, it's not natural behavior to just go wherever she may feel like it. Obviously, going to the bathroom is the best place for this to happen. This is what she needs to learn and understand, as well as realize that it's a safe space for her to do her business.

When she starts following you into the bathroom, encourage her curiosity and start the potty-training process with her, there and then, by educating her on what's happening. Also keep her interests when it comes to bathroom activities. This may mean that you won't have any alone time in the bathroom for a while.

Let Her Observe

Whenever you or your spouse go to the bathroom, let your daughter observe what's happening. If she's at her grandparents house, let her follow, as long as they're comfortable with it, so that she can see that everyone does this. You may have to be careful that she doesn't follow a friend into the bathroom, or a stranger if you're eating out at a restaurant, for example.

While her dad may be uncomfortable with her following him into the bathroom, this will also allow her to understand that there are differences between boys and girls. Dad's also have their part to play in potty-training, and it will also help that it's a team effort that can celebrate her success as she goes through the potty-training. There will, however, be more of an emphasis on mom's toilet habits.

You are going to have to explain to her why dad stands and mom sits, as she may find this to be somewhat confusing. You also don't want her to try and imitate dad and stand over the potty when she's going through her potty-training. She'll start to understand that going to the toilet is a natural process and that there's nothing to be scared of.

Be prepared for a million questions. Some of them will be asked more than once, especially when it comes to the anatomical differences between girls and boys. You may not know where the toilet paper goes to, or exactly how the toilet works, but there will be no right or wrong answer to give her.

Encourage Curiosity

Every child has a natural curiosity, and being open and encouraging this curiosity is important when it comes to potty-training. It may be very uncomfortable, and a tad embarrassing, if she's trying to get a good look at you or your spouse while you're taking care of business. What you want to happen is for her to imitate what you're doing, though, so that she can be comfortable when she needs to do this.

You'll be very surprised at the questions and statements that can come out of their little mouths. If your child is an early bloomer and is mastering potty-training, then she may not be able to string a whole sentence together. Just let her watch and copy.

While you may be left feeling shy, as your child stares at you while you're doing your business, it's important that your child doesn't feel embarrassed or ashamed for watching. Eventually, when they're using the potty they won't give any of your bits a second thought. Children learn how to do things by mimicking us, their parents, and this goes on for the first few years of their lives. To be successful with potty-training, let them imitate you often.

Get Her Excited About It

The best way to keep a child's attention is to make something super exciting. The more excited she is about the toilet the more interest she'll show and the more she'll learn. So how do you turn an ordinary toilet into a magical interest factory?

You can try:

- Let her place brightly colored stickers on the toilet.
- Let her decorate and bedazzle her potty or toilet seat attachment.
- Get her a toilet buddy that also loves to use the potty. This can be a doll or fluffy toy.
- Create a sticker chart and let her help to decorate it.
- You can also read to her while she's just sitting in the potty.

When you go and buy the potty, take her with you and tell her you're going to buy a very special potty, just for her. This way she won't be disappointed when she doesn't get a doll. While you have her with you, get her interested in the potty and see what she's drawn to and what she'd find to be comfortable.

While you're at the store, tell her it's time that she gets her own big-girl panties. Then, let her choose what she wants. If she's drawn to cartoon characters from Frozen, or she wants butterflies, then let her have those. You want her to be so excited that she can't wait to wear them. You'll have to choose neutral and plain panties for her as well. As mentioned previously, be sure to get her up to 20-30 pairs. This will come in handy if she has an accident.

Don't hide the panties or the potty when you get home. Instead, leave them out for her to see. Tell her that in a week she can start wearing them and in the days leading up to the potty-training, let her decorate her potty.

If she's determined to wear the panties sooner than that, take a couple of pairs out for her and let her run around the house in them. This will help her to get comfortable with the change, but be prepared for accidents as well. The rest you can tell her are for when she starts the training.

Have you noticed how kids get excited over the holidays? There's the build up of seeing the decorations and then the countdown to Christmas Eve. Then finally it's Christmas morning, and they just can't contain their excitement! For the days leading up to the potty-training, you want to try and create that type of excitement; this is the day for her big-girl training.

Parental Preparation

So now your daughter is telling all her stuffed toys that she's going to be a big girl soon, and she's all excited. You've prepared everything for her, double-checked that it's all ready. Now all that's left to do is the parental preparation. Next to planning your wedding day, this can be the second most stressful time of your life, but it doesn't have to be and it won't be. You'll be organized for this and you're going to anticipate and expect speed bumps and accidents to happen.

You can plan and make your meals in advance for the weekend, so that all you have to do is take them out of the freezer and pop them into the oven. If you feel the need to prepare a hiccup kit (Pee or poop accident kit), then by all means get the gloves, buckets and sponges ready.

Schedule the Weekend

Plan the weekend in advance so that you can let your friends and loved ones know that you're not going to be available. Sit with your partner and see which weekend will best suit you both and mark that on the calendar. Make sure that you have everything that you'll need for that weekend, this includes snacks for you and your partner.

Once you have set the date and there's nothing happening but potty-training that weekend, you need to make sure that it won't be pushed back or cancelled. So you'll need to plan around school and sport schedules, work schedules as well as social schedules.

You'll want this weekend to have no interruptions. Family and friends will know that you're potty-training and if need be, you can get the grandparents to hold you accountable. It's not necessary, but some people find it to be helpful and this will also mean there's no wiggle room for procrastination.

It's also important to remember that life happens and things that are beyond your control could come up. You could come down with a terrible cold or an emergency could happen. You don't just want to back out of the potty-training because you're "not in the right frame of mind" or "you're not ready," or because there's a Game of Thrones rerun marathon that you don't want to miss.

Have someone that you can be accountable to and that you can also vent to if you're feeling frustrated over the weekend. This offers a lifeline to someone that you trust who can help put things into perspective if it's needed.

Get the Other Kids Out for the Weekend

If you have an older child who has gone through potty-training, it may be a good idea to send them to a friend's house or to their grandparents (if that's an option). This will mean that your little girl will have no distractions when it comes to her potty-training over the weekend.

While you don't want your other child to feel as though they're not special to you, you may want to make their weekend fun as well. So, what do you do if your other child just wants to stay at home? You can't force them to leave, but you can let them know that their sibling is going to be potty-training and that they can get involved if they like. Their help could be invaluable as well. This will allow the older sibling the chance to be the big sister or brother who can teach the young one a thing or two and that's not sprinkled in mischief.

This may require a little more planning on your part. But if your little girl looks up to her older sibling, it could come in handy to have them around to help show the young one the ropes.

Cheerleading and Tracking Success

Some children will respond well to verbal praise while others may not fully understand what's going on. So when you praise them, you may have to change the tone of your voice, facial expression and body language. We all change the tones of our voices when speaking to young children, you know, the baby voice you can't help but do. Children respond to this because they can understand tone of voice more than the words we're saying.

You've seen how children watch and respond to our facial expressions. When we pull funny faces, they erupt into giggles. They are also aware of when we frown or don't look happy. So when you're potty-training your little girl, you may want to be more animated with your facial expressions and change your tone of voice when praising her.

To become your child's potty-training cheerleader, you can be as creative as you want to be. There are some things that you can do that will encourage your little girl to make progress with her potty-training, like:

- Creating a celebrating dance and song
- Make a funny noise that's followed by action, like raising your hands and going, "Whoop, Whoop!"
- Sounds that make potty-training fun (dad's love making "passing gas" noises)
- Rewrite the lyrics to your girl's favorite show tune to include potty-training

Every time your child uses the potty or has a small victory, play the song, make the sound or do the dance. If this gets your little girl laughing hysterically, then she'll want to recreate the moment so that you'll do it again. This will keep the potty-training fun and exciting.

I understand that some people aren't comfortable singing or dancing, even if it's in front of the children or your spouse. I was extremely shy growing up. It took me what seems like a lifetime to get comfortable enough around my family to dance, sing or behave like a clown. If you're similar to me, then maybe look at using squeaky toys that can help you create a celebratory sound.

Stock Up on Supplies

Before the big-girl potty-training weekend, make sure that you've stocked up on everything that you'll need or want. You don't want to have to run to the store quickly because you forgot something. This will allow you to give your little girl your full undivided attention and you won't miss out on any moments of success.

Create a shopping list of everything that you may need, so you can tick it off when you get it. Stock up on milk, coffee and snacks as you're going to be home for three days. You can also make sure that you've got the following organized for the weekend:

Meals

Can you imagine what it would have felt like if you had missed your little girls first step because you were cooking in the kitchen? Well, you don't want to miss the opportunity when she uses the potty by herself for the first time either. You can prepare meals during the week and freeze them until you're ready to use them on the weekend. This will free up a lot of time, since you won't have to spend 30 minutes (or more) preparing and then cooking the food. Not to mention having to clean the kitchen and wash the dishes later.

You'll want to make sure that all meals have less processed food and that they contain healthy foods that will stimulate your little girls bowel movements. In order for effective potty-training to take place, you need to create the matter in your child's stomach to make it happen. It's better to have too much food that you can save as a meal for the next week, than too little food where you'll end up cooking. This will also take the worry out of what to prepare and when.

Plan the foods ahead of time and start changing your child's diet two days before the potty-training is to start. This will get their bodily functions working so you won't have to wait too long before getting started.

If you can, try to stick to high-fiber foods like:

- Fresh fruit and vegetables
- Coconut and avocado to get things moving
- Prune pouches
- Bran cereal or oatmeal.

Snacks

You want to give your little girl a lot of fiber and a lot of fluids to drink. The fiber will stimulate her digestive system, which will allow for many opportunities to use the potty. But with this comes accidents as well. Fiber will help to soften her poop, as well as bulk it up, which will make the whole process easier on your little girl.

Here are some ideas for high-fiber snacks for the weekend:

- Dried fruit (Prunes are great for this)
- Apples and pears or similar grainy fruits
- Granola bars
- Popcorn (be careful of kernels)
- Berries (it doesn't matter if they're strawberries or blueberries)
- Whole grain crackers

Stay away from foods that would bind, as this can make your girl constipated. You'll also have to watch her dairy intake as that can make her constipated too, so don't give her too much ice-cream or milk.

You can give your daughter fruit juice or water to drink, and I found it helpful to leave a sippy cup in every room. I would also encourage my child to drink more frequently, so that they'd have to use the toilet more often.

Try and avoid drinks that contain high levels of sugar. If you're giving her fruit juice, try to make sure that it's 100% juice. If you want her to only drink water, you could try adding a few drops of water flavoring, like some fruit juice, to encourage her to drink more.

Cleaning Supplies

I mentioned having a cleaning kit earlier in the book, and this will come in handy. There are going to be accidents around the house. Remember that this may embarrass her, as well. As difficult as it may be, try not show your frustration. You'll need cleaning supplies close on hand. You don't want to make it obvious that they're close by, as we don't want her to think that you cleaning up after her is the new normal or that you're just waiting for her to have an accident. What you'll need:

- A plastic bucket
- Cleaning cloths
- Deodorizing cleaning solution
- Bath towel for when she needs it

If you have any carpets that aren't glued down that you're worried about, roll them up and put them out the way. This will help to make your house potty-safe. The next chapter is going to take you through the processes of Day 1 Potty-Training. Read through it again the night before so that you're comfortable with what the day entails.

Chapter 4:

Day 1

The big day has arrived, and we're about to start potty-training! You've got everything you need to do the potty-training and you're raring to go. One last look at the checklist as you should have:

- ❏ No activities planned outside of the potty-training
- ❏ Arrangements have been made for your other children
- ❏ All meals have been prepared in advance
- ❏ Activity schedule in place to keep your daughter busy
- ❏ Potty chair or potty seat are in the bathroom
- ❏ Big-girl panties are stacked and ready for use
- ❏ Drinking cups filled and placed around the house
- ❏ High-fiber snacks are ready to be eaten
- ❏ Check with spouse to make sure you're still on the same page
- ❏ Message loved ones and let them know you're only available for emergencies
- ❏ Potty-training success chart up
- ❏ Cleaning kit strategically positioned so you can grab it quickly

If you've ticked everything off, then all that you need to do is start the day. We're going to go through this step-by-step so you know what your day ahead looks like. This will help you to set the tone for the day, but bear in mind that this is also flexible. You may find that you race through step 1 and step 2 only to find that your little girl is hungry or distracted by the dog. Feed your princess, give the dog a bone and move onto step 3.

You'll need to make sure that you get through all the steps in the day, and if you get through them all and it's not bed time, you can repeat the steps. Getting your child to repeat the steps twice will help to reinforce the training. Go about your normal daily activities in between the potty-training steps and encourage your daughter to drink and play like she normally would.

Try not to leave the house on day one, as this will mean that you have to put a diaper on your daughter (or she's going to have to leave the house without a diaper which will mean risking an accident). This would be embarrassing for her, and she may not want to continue with the potting training.

If you want your child to be diaper-free, then you have to be committed to the process. There can't be any half measures over the course of the next three days, as this will make the training less effective. The steps have been designed to achieve having your little girl be potty-trained by the end of the weekend. This is laying the foundation of good toilet habits. If you change the steps or leave steps out of the process, this could have a negative impact or your child may decide that she's not going to go along with it.

Customize the steps so that your child feels comfortable, but it's important that you follow them as closely as possible so that the training is effective. Throw in something that your daughter loves and would be interested in, for each step. If you're working on step 3, get her excited if need be, grab her doll and put panties on her as well. This way they can potty-traintogether. Whatever you can do to make sure that your child is engaged and excited about the training will help.

There isn't anybody in the world who can speak your daughter's language better than you! You understand her personality, habits, fears, moods and what motivates her. Be creative and make it a fun experience, there's no reason why potty-training has to be difficult or a lengthy process.

Play with your daughter, have a tea party, color with her or even read to her. If you have a bit of a backyard, why not plant strawberries or flowers? Do some arts and crafts and start a finger painting. You want the time to be spent having fun and keeping your daughter in a positive frame of mind. Just remember to keep her drinking and nibbling on those high-fiber snacks. You can even watch a movie with popcorn to end the day off in a fun way.

The potty-training process is straightforward and easy to follow and all you need to do is fit this into your day. I'll give an explanation of each step so that you can see why it's better to follow the process. There'll be some tips and advice for you as well. These tips I have found in my own personal experience to be very useful, and they've even led to more victories over the 3-day training.

Both you and your spouse need to stay positive, calm and patient as this will be a big factor to the success of the method. Your girl will be watching you and she'll know if you're not genuinely excited and motivated over the weekend. In order to keep her excited and motivated, you both have to be. Now I understand that life happens and arguments can happen at any moment between two people, but remember that this will hinder the effectiveness of the training. Your child will be concerned about what is happening and the feelings that she's sensing, which could have an impact on her potty-training.

Step 1 - First You Need to Start Your Day

The day begins with you! You're the most important part of your daughter's life; she looks up to you, she learns from you, she's reassured by you. In a nutshell, you and your spouse are her world! This weekend she'll be following your lead the whole weekend and for every step. Start your day with something that will set the happy tone as she'll notice this almost immediately when you wake her up.

Sing in the shower, dance your way to the kitchen for your morning coffee, you can even take 30 minutes to read the newspaper before waking your little princess up. Do what your morning routine normally entails before waking her up. This will help you get a head start on the day.

I love being organized and sometimes it may seem like I overly prepare, but I found that preparing my home for potty-training saved time, money and loads of frustration, especially when there were accidents. This will also make cleaning up accidents easier.

In the morning you should take some time for yourself, go through what needs to be done and make sure that you've got everything that you need for the day ahead. Carving some quiet time out for you is important, especially as you're going to be spending a lot of your time with your little one over the next three days.

You can choose if you want to have breakfast as a family; then you can prepare it and then get your little girl up. Start the day off with a high-fiber breakfast and you can start step 2 at the breakfast table!

Step 2 - Get Her Excited About It

You want to get your daughter excited about the day ahead and start with celebrating the fact that she can put her "big-girl" panties on. Let her choose her outfit, but it would be better if she wears a dress as this will make the first day of potty-training easy. Some parents will put the panties on with a T-shirt and let their girls run around the house like that.

Once you've had a healthy, high-fiber breakfast, go to her room and start with getting rid of her diapers. You'll need to make show of getting rid of the diapers in a positive way and get her involved as you don't want her thinking that she's going to miss them. You can even get her stuffed toys involved. Let her toss some of the diapers into the bin or on the floor.

Make a fuss over her and how she's dressed for the day! Think about how you feel when someone pays you a compliment on an outfit you're wearing. It's important that there's lots of praise and excitement. Remember to use your body language, facial expressions and tone of voice. You can reassure her with lots of hugs and kisses as well. You'll have to be more animated and speak in a "baby" voice as she'll pick up on how you're saying things versus what you're saying.

Now that the diapers have been tossed out, you've praised her for being such a big girl, it's time to get her new toilet. If she's picked this out herself she'll be excited to use it. If she doesn't seem too excited about it this time round, you can always let her decorate it or get one of her toys to sit in it. You can get very creative about how to get her excited about the potty again.

Now let's get started on step 3!

Step 3 - Explain the Basics

Your daughter needs to understand that if she goes in her big-girl underpants that it's very different from her diaper. One way you can do this is to show her that water flows through it by actually holding a pair of panties under a tap, so she can see and feel them. You'll also need to tell her that when she needs to make a wee, she needs to tell you before this happens.

Now show her how her big-girl panties work, this way she knows that she needs to pull them down before she makes a wee. You can have a couple of trial runs of her pulling them up and down, so that you can be sure that she can do this. This will also help when she needs to hop onto the potty as she's already done this a couple of times. It is very possible that by the time she needs to use the potty, she may have forgotten how to pull her panties down. Repetition is the key to making this stick and needs to be done in a fun way. However, once she's discovered that she can take them off...well, she may take them off and run wild and free through the house.

Using one of her dolls, show her how to sit in the potty and explain that this is where she'll make the wee or the poo. You can put a diaper in the potty to layer it as she already associates this with wee and poo and tell her that when she needs to go, she just needs to pull down her panties and go on top of the diaper.

I used this technique with my middle child and it worked like a charm. He knew that the diaper was there for his wees and poos, and he'd go and settle himself on his potty and do his business on the diaper like he needed to. This also helped with the cleaning of the potty and I would just throw away the diaper and put a new one down for him. Once he got the hang of going to the potty, I removed the diaper, and he just had a look, turned around and used the potty without it.

You want your child to recognize when she needs to go and link the feeling of wanting to wee to the action of peeing in the potty. This is tricky and you'll have to ask her when she may want to go, but she may also just go in her panties as this has been normal for her. Patience will be required. You also want to limit how many times you ask her about when she wants to go; she may end up thinking that she needs to when she doesn't.

Give her some space as well. You don't need to hover over her. You want her to feel when she needs to go. Keep her fueled with snacks and beverages and wait patiently while you enjoy some family activities.

Step 4 - Be Attentive

There's a fine balance between hovering and being attentive. This can be tricky in and of itself. Should your little girl have an accident, you'd need to grab her quickly and put her on the potty, so she can finish her business on the potty. You'll also have to make sure that you're not coming across as aggressive or panicked when this happens.

Your child isn't going to want to have accidents, and she's going to be embarrassed by what's happened, but it's the quickest way for her to recognize how to feel when she needs to go. This will happen a couple of times but, I can assure you that she'll understand the feeling of wanting to go a lot quicker than if you're prompting her to go.

You also can't leave her where she is when she's having an accident, as this will give her a mixed signal and confuse her about where she actually needs to go. Watch to see if she's looking for a place to hide as this could be a sign of her wanting to relieve herself.

It's important that you don't leave her to take a nap or play with her toys and think that she's going to tug on your sleeve when she wants to go. She's not at that stage. Your little girl can't do this without you, so you have to keep a watchful eye on her. Your job is to get her to the potty as quickly as you can when she starts to have an accident.

Yes, you're going to end up with a trail of wee over the floor, you're going to be washing underwear and hopefully, you won't find any poop surprises behind your couch, (this happened to a friend of mine when her toddler disappeared, removed her panties and did her business). While you may have to keep a watchful eye on her, and sprint across the room, this is the most effective way to get your child potty-trained.

After a couple of accidents, the link between the brain and the body will kick-in, and she'll start to recognize when she needs to go, instead of relying on either you or spouse to take her.

Things to Remember

Spending this much time with your little one and having to keep a watch can be exhausting! You're going to get frustrated. There are going to be times when you question your sanity and you're not going to love having to clean up another accident. If you're asking yourself if it's worth it, know that the answer isa resounding yes!

Once you've got the foundation in place, you've got through the process with love, patience, sheer determination and lots of toilet paper, you'll see the results.

When you're feeling rough and you want to throw in the towel, remember these things:

Accidents Are Going to Happen

As sure as the day is long, you can expect your daughter to have a couple of accidents on the first day. Sometimes your child will have to go through a number of accidents in one day and this could be what gets the penny to drop. Sometimes it only takes two or three accidents and your daughter will realize what is happening.

Whatever the number of accidents, it's an important part of the learning curve. The three things that are needed here are:

- Focus
- Patience
- Calm

It's of the utmost importance that you don't respond out of frustration or anger at any time, when an accident happens. You want to react calmly, with love and understanding as you're going to have to reassure your little one when they're embarrassed. You'll need to pick her up, dust her off, motivate her and let her start again each time there's an accident, knowing that at the end of it all, she'll gain confidence and will use the potty.

Praise Her When She Does It Right

You're going to have to nudge your daughter in the right way, so every now and then just say, "Let me know when you need to go." When she does let you know, your heart will feel like it's going to burst with pride. You may even feel like you want to cry, but before you do, get her to the potty! Praise her all the way to the potty, let the cheerleader in you loose! Raise your hands in the air and "Whoop, Whoop" her.

You need to be consistent with your praise as well, and make sure that every time she gets it right, the same level of enthusiasm is there. Even if she just misses the mark, praise her with a bit less enthusiasm for almost getting it right and tell her that next time she'll get it right! Positive reinforcement the whole way! Remind her to tell you when she needs to go and, if you have the chart up, let her stick the stars or stickers on to it.

Do a dance while she's sticking her sticker to her chart. Praise her for the progress she has made. When she does finally manage to wee or poo in the potty, that's when you raise the ceiling on the house! It doesn't matter if it's a trickle or a drop, she needs all the positive reinforcement she can get. This will also encourage her to go to the potty again to do her business.

At every point where she is successful, praise her and increase the enthusiasm and the praise as she gets closer to letting you know when she needs the potty and when she uses the potty.

Be Careful How You Say Things

You don't want to ask your little princess if she needs to go to the toilet or if she needs to wee or poo. Rather prompt her by saying, "Do you need to wee" or "Tell me when you want to use the potty." This helps your child to become more self-aware. She'll be able to figure it out and make her own decision about needing to go to the potty. If you keep asking her, she could go when she doesn't need to, just to please you. Or she could feel like she's being pressured and not do anything at all.

This allows her the freedom to actually feel what her body is doing, as opposed to thinking that's what her body is doing. The link between the brain and the body is being created, and she'll become aware that the feeling is linked to her needing to go and relieve herself.

Remember to use positive tones in your voice, positive body language and facial expressions as you don't want to confuse her by sending mixed signals. Especially if you remind her after she had an accident. You don't want her feeling like she has done something wrong. If she feels like she's constantly doing something wrong, she could withhold her poop. This will just lead to constipation and the weekend will be over.

You're encouraging her to come to you and tell you when she's ready to go, without being nagged.

Make Sure Your Daughter Is Ready Before Beginning

You're probably in bed, under the covers feeling slightly nervous about the first day of the potty-training. Run through the signs that your daughter has been showing consistently, so that you know that she's ready for the potty-training. It's very important that she's ready both physically and developmentally for the training. If you've gone over the signs, and you're 100% sure that she's not ready, postpone the training.

However, if you've been seeing the signs consistently, and more than one sign, then go ahead with the training. As much as we want our girls to be potty-trained, it's not a process that can be forced or rushed into. You shouldn't potty-train your child just because you want to or you think she should be potty-trained. Rushing into potty-training can have long-lasting negative and deeply scarring effects on your child, if they're not ready for potty-training (Dewar, 2010).

It can also cause a lot of frustration and anger in a parent when the child isn't ready, and they're not getting the results they want. This frustration and anger can have devastating effects on your child. She may feel she has done something wrong, and she'll sense that you're angry with her. This can hamper any future potty-training attempts since she may associate the anger and frustration with the potty.

Once you're 1000 percent sure, go ahead with day 1 potty-training.

When the first day of potty-training is over, flop into bed and get a good night's rest. Skim through the section on "Day Two," which is covered in the next chapter, so that it's fresh in your mind when you wake up in the morning.

Chapter 5:

Days Two and Three

Well done on making it through day one! You may be feeling ready for day two, or you might be feeling overwhelmed and worried about how it's going to go. Don't worry - you're a third of the way through the process already!

Remember to take care of yourself before your daughter wakes up. Take a refreshing shower and have a good breakfast, and if you can, run through the schedule with your spouse one more time. Yesterday was the beginning of this new adventure. Today will be about continuing with normal life and allowing your daughter to begin recognizing what her body is telling her.

I have a tip for beginning the day. Make sure your daughter has a good, high-fiber breakfast with something to drink. Take her straight to the potty when she's done. She will most likely remember what this is all about, and once breakfast is done she will probably need to go very soon after anyway.

Once you're off to that good start, briefly remind your daughter of how well she did the day before and encourage her to try to do the same today. If you start the day with positive reinforcement, it will set the tone for a good day ahead (Souders, 2019). Remind her to let you know today when she needs to pee or poop.

It's important that you have enough to keep your daughter busy during the day today. Although we will be venturing outside at some point, you will be spending a lot of time at home and boredom can lead to grumpy children. We want her to be as happy as possible!

So, step number one - like yesterday, start off your own morning before your little girl wakes up. When she's up, make sure to offer positive reinforcement and get her excited about the day ahead.

Here's what you need to keep in mind throughout the day...

Steps to Follow Through the Day

Although the aim is to keep things fun and relaxed, it's important to know what you need to be doing as the day goes. Remember, we have a goal here - to get your little girl to go potty. Everything you do this weekend should be with that in mind.

Thankfully, the schedule is still flexible and as long as you regularly check in on these few actions you should be a-okay.

Keep Her Hydrated

Hydration is always important, but it's also quite key when it comes to potty-training. More juice equals more pee, and that means more opportunities for her to realize that her body is trying to tell her something.

Stick to natural fruit juice or as healthy a drink as you can. Please don't feed your child sugary soft drinks throughout the weekend - not only will this make for very bad dental health, but mom and dad will be dealing with a hyped-up child who will most likely have a sugar crash later in the day.

If your little girl isn't drinking much, you can try some creative fun things to get her to drink more. Try:

- Challenging her to drink her juice faster than you can drink yours.
- Playing her favorite game and letting the winner have a sip of juice every time (and then let her win)!

- Get her favorite cups or sippy bottles, fill some with water and some with juice. Then go around your house and leave them in spots where she can reach them. You can even make a game out of her drinking from the various cups.

Keep Her Eating

As well as drinking, you need to feed your daughter as much as you can throughout the day. Don't "force" her to eat, but make sure she is getting in enough high-fiber snacks to stimulate a bowel movement.

Just like with the drinks, make sure what you're feeding her is good, healthy food. This weekend should not be filled with chips, chocolate, and sugary foods. There are plenty of very healthy and still tasty snacks that will do the trick, and she'll be quite happy with them.

That doesn't mean you can't reward her with a small bit of chocolate or a packet of chips. But she will be eating more over this weekend than usual, so it's up to you to make sure she doesn't overindulge in unhealthy things. You also really don't want to end up trying to potty-train a child with an upset stomach.

A snack and a glass of juice every hour or every 30 minutes should do the trick. You will probably have to eat and drink with her, so be warned! There should be no calorie-counting over the weekend. Just keep the snacks small. Remember you don't need to feed her big snacks. Share a packet of popcorn between the three of you, or have a few slices of cheese and some dried fruit.

Keep an Eye on Her

In between making sure that your daughter is eating and drinking, keep your eyes peeled for signs that she needs to go to the potty.

Even though she knows she should be telling you, it may take a couple of tries before she gets it right, so you'll need to keep an eye on her and notice any signs early on to avoid an accident.

If a pee or poop surprises her, it's important that you don't become angry or annoyed. Patience is the key. Offer positive reinforcement, always!

If you do notice signs, don't rush your little girl off to the toilet. Just gently remind her to let you know if she needs to go. This isn't nagging, but it does offer a gentle reminder of something that she may have forgotten.

If she says no, then don't argue with her, no matter what signs you see! This is about allowing her the space to understand what her body is saying, and if it requires a couple of accidents to get that right, then so be it.

Some common signs include:

- Squatting
- Flatulence
- Restlessness
- Dancing around or bouncing on the spot
- Crossing her legs tightly
- Grabbing or holding her crotch area
- Trying to pull her underwear off

Don't automatically assume one of these signs means she's aching to go. If she's watching her favorite TV show, she could simply be getting excited and bouncing around a little. If you're sitting in a room with two parents and pets, that musty flatulent smell could just as easily be a dog…or dad.

Be aware, be discerning, and be patient.

Get Her to the Bathroom Quickly (When She Needs to Go)

When you get that go-ahead to take her to the potty, don't dawdle. Get her there as quickly as possible. Although she's getting better at understanding her body, she's still developing and can't hold it in for very long.

Either lead her to the potty or pick her up and take her there. Help her to take her panties off and get in the right position, and do what she needs to do.

If she begins to have an accident, remain calm and do not get angry. It may be instinctual to show some annoyance, but you will need to actively work at keeping your cool.

If you can, move her to the potty, so she can finish there. If you can't, that's also okay. Don't be upset, and keep encouraging and supporting. Don't make her feel like she did something wrong. She will already know that next time, she should be more careful.

If she did make it to the potty before she let it go, praise her! Reward her with a sticker on her chart or a small toy, whatever you feel is appropriate.

Make Sure There Are No Distractions

As I'm sure you can see, you'll need to be quite attentive during the day with your little girl. It's very important that you stay away from distractions during these three days. Of course, you need to keep your child busy, but avoiding distractions is more for parents than it is for the child. Whether she's busy or not, she's going to need to go potty. But you need to be ready every moment for it to happen, so you can be supportive and help her reach this milestone.

Life carries on, no matter whether or not you're potty-training your daughter, but you will need to avoid the temptation of social media, visits, long phone calls, or your own hobbies.

Every minute of this weekend should be about your daughter, and teaching her this skill. You've already let everyone know that you'll be unavailable, so they should be respectful enough to honor that and allow you and your family space.

I know emergencies do happen, and there's no avoiding that. If you need to take a call, or make coffee, or step outside so you can cry without your daughter seeing you, then do so. Just keep it brief. Don't leave your daughter playing with her dolls while you scroll through Instagram.

Remember your child will also probably need to take a nap sometime during the day. You can use this time to catch up on things you may need or want to do.

Things to Keep in Mind

This weekend is about teaching your child to use the toilet quickly and effectively. But with this habit comes other important hygiene habits that they should also learn. The earlier we teach children these things, the quicker they become ingrained.

Good toilet hygiene is essential. Although learning to pee and poop in the right place is basically what potty-training is about, none of us want our children walking out of the bathroom and grabbing a sandwich if they've just emptied their poop into the big toilet and forgotten to wash their hands.

We all want our children to be healthy! That's what hygiene is about. Now is the perfect time to begin teaching your little girl how to keep good toilet hygiene. That way, the habit of peeing or pooping in the toilet, flushing and washing their hands will be instilled together, as a sort of toilet hygiene package. You don't want your daughter to be that person everyone raises their eyebrows at, when she walks out the bathroom stall and leaves without so much as glancing at the faucet.

These habits are as important as the actual potty-training. Teaching them together creates an association in your daughter's mind that is very hard to break once it's there.

Hand Washing

Hand washing is honestly very easy to do. Do not neglect it! It's essential to keep healthy, and we all want our children to be healthy.

First, you need to lead by example. Especially if your daughter has been following you to the toilet and watching you, it's imperative that she sees you do this action every single time. Not once or twice, not when you feel like it - every single time after you do your business.

If she sees you brushing it off, you're not going to be able to get her to believe that it's an important action. If it's something you struggle with, maybe you and your daughter can get into the habit together! Either way, you need to make sure you consciously do this every single time you go.

Make a big deal of it. Lather the soap on your hands, rub it through your fingers, and up your wrists. If you want to, you can even get your daughter her own soap. Maybe a princess soap, to get her extra excited about washing her hands!

Most children will need a step in order to reach the basin. Make sure that the step is sturdy and won't slip on the floor. This is for your own peace of mind as well as to make your little one feel safe and secure! Even though you will be with her every time she washes her hands, eventually she will have to do it by herself.

It could be a good idea to place a rubber mat underneath the step to keep it as sturdy as possible. Don't worry about how your bathroom looks! This is about safety, and it's a hugely important aspect.

Wiping

Wiping may seem like such a simple action, but there is a right way and a less right way to do it. Although wiping from back to front is not necessarily incorrect (it still does the job), it can increase the chances of infection.

Even though your little girl has been watching you, she's not going to notice every detail in vivid clarity. You will need to explain to her exactly how to wipe, and it's a good idea to instill the "front-to-back" thing in her from the start. If she learns the other way around, it can be nearly impossible to change later on.

You can show her how to do it by standing behind her, placing the toilet paper in her hand, and guiding her hand to wipe the right way. This should do the trick, and you can check on her to make sure she's doing it the way you showed her.

"Front to back" is important for both peeing and pooping. When she pees, she needs to be wiping the moisture away without wiping bacteria from the back right onto her sensitive bits. This can open the door for nasty infections, including urinary tract and kidney infections.

As for pooping, the same applies. She should be wiping in the opposite direction to keep bacteria away from other areas. Although she is going to be bathed, this is an important habit to instill in order to promote good health. Bacteria can make a home quickly, and bathing won't always necessarily get rid of them.

Imitation

Your little girl learns a lot by watching and imitating you (Meltzoff, 1999). You've taken the time to allow her to come to the bathroom with you in preparation for this weekend, and that shouldn't stop now.

She may see this experience in a new light now that she is doing it herself. Remember, this imitation thing isn't just about the toilet - it's about flushing, hand washing, drying, and cleaning. Now is also a great time to teach her to clean up after herself.

Positive Reinforcement

You can't use too much positive reinforcement over this weekend. It may get tiresome for you, but she will appreciate and learn from it. Use it when:

- She lets you know that she needs to go
- She gets to the potty in time to do her thing
- She can pull her panties down by herself
- She positions herself correctly on the potty
- She pees or poops in the potty (even if she misses slightly)
- She flushes when she's finished
- She washes her hands with soap
- She dries her hands after washing them

Getting Out of the House

If things are going well, you can make short trips out of the house with your daughter on day two and three. You should:

Prepare

It's a good idea to include a trip in your schedule from the beginning. If you don't feel your child is ready for it, you can always leave it. But it's important to be prepared, so that if you do decide to take a little trip you're as ready as can be for what may happen.

It's not a good idea to do something that is going to be long-winded, like shopping, visiting friends, or a long car trip. You should be out for 20 to 30 minutes, and no longer.

Prepare yourself for this little excursion by:

- Choosing the right kind of outing
- Taking an extra set of clothes along

- Taking clean-up supplies with you
- Try and make sure that your child won't end up in a situation where she could be embarrassed

Remember your positive reinforcement, even when you're out of the house!

Be Quick

If you're nervous about being out of the house, try 10 or 15 minutes in the backyard first, away from the potty. If it goes well, both you and your little girl will have more confidence and you can up the backyard visit to 20 to 30 minutes.

Don't be out for less than that, though. 5 minutes outside before rushing back in is not at all enough time to allow the process to take place. You'll need at least 10 minutes, but closer to 20 is better.

Be careful where you choose to go if you're leaving the property. Away from roads is always best, and somewhere you'll be able to leave when you need to in order to get your little girl back home.

If she tells you she needs to go, get her to the closest toilet. If she has an accident, clean her up, give her some encouragement, and get home. This may take a few tries to get it right.

Be Calm

Leaving the house with an undiapered child can be a scary prospect! But it's important not to get freaked out by this step. It can be rough, waiting for an accident to happen but fervently hoping that it doesn't.

I urge you to not rush through this step! For some parents, it's so daunting that they simply skip it entirely, but it's an important part of the process and of your daughter's learningcurve.

Nobody wants their child to poop in public, of course. But your confidence in your child is extremely important in this step. Even if you're expecting an accident at any minute, you need to act natural and show confidence in your child. Just be normal, and your daughter will feel at ease.

If your little girl tells you she needs to go, be calm, give her some praise and get her to the closest toilet. If she has an accident, stay just as calm, keep your words neutral but be encouraging. Clean her up and make sure there's no chance of her being even more embarrassed, for example, by making a big deal of it and strangers noticing.

If you aren't sure what to do to get out of the house, why not try some of these ideas:

- Take the dogs for a run around the block or in the park

- Spend some time playing Frisbee or kicking a ball in the park

- Garden work is a great out-of-the-house-but-not-too-far-away activity

- Visit the store briefly if you need to grab something quick

- Pop in to see a friend for a quick visit

Chapter 6:

After the Three Days

Parents, I know it can be extremely tempting to put in a monumental effort for three days and then put it behind you and forget it ever happened. I understand! Those three days are not fun and games for parents. Your daughter may adore being waited on hand and foot for an entire weekend, but it can be very taxing on the parents involved.

But if you immediately put it out of your mind and pretend it never happened, it will be infinitely harder for your little girl to carry on doing the same thing effectively. You need to be actively involved in encouraging and reinforcing this process, even after the first three days.

Remember, just because your child can use their own potty at home, or even the potty seat, that doesn't necessarily mean they're completely and fully potty-trained. Daycare, for example, may be difficult for her because it's not the same toilet. It's out of her comfort zone, and will take some getting used to.

Going forward after the initial three days can be a challenge. It's very likely there will still be accidents in the weeks and months to come, and there will be plenty of opportunity for frustration and annoyance to pop up. Resist, parents!

The weekend comes with a flood of different feelings. You'll have had moments of excitement, anticipation, happiness, frustration and defeat. But at the end of it, you should be brimming with pride and happiness that your little princess has made such amazing progress.

This is the attitude that you'll need to cling to for dear life in the upcoming weeks and months. Remember all the progress she's made and how far she's come! If she keeps going with just as much success, then you've done a great job. If there are a few accidents along the way, it's normal, to be expected, and nothing at all to stress about.

If it so happens that your little girl regresses to the point of needing a diaper again, don't worry. It's rare, but it does happen, and it doesn't mean you've failed, or she's failed. It simply means you need to dig a little deeper before trying again. Regression can be triggered by certain things, and once you know what the cause is, it can almost always be rectified quickly.

Going forward, you need to stay actively involved in the process.

Reinforcement

Even though you'll be going back to the real world, where parents have to work and children have to go back to daycare, it's essential to be observant and keep reinforcing what she's learned over the weekend. If your child spends most of her time at daycare, it could be a great idea to chat to her daycare teachers and ask them to reinforce what she's learned, if there's an opportunity.

Evenings and weekends may be the only time busy parents have to reinforce these behaviors, but it's important that you don't let it slide. Take time to observe, practice, and reinforce what your child learned over those three days. Use the same techniques that your daughter responded well to over the weekend. If she really liked the sticker chart approach, keep using that until the concept is well and truly reinforced.

Perhaps the most important thing is to continue to offer love, encouragement, and positive reinforcement. Just because you're not spending the entire weekend waiting for her to announce that she needs to go, this doesn't mean that your praise and encouragement isn't necessary and very appreciated! If you suddenly start acting like her going potty on her own isn't important, she's likely to be rather confused, not to mention a little upset.

Encourage, encourage, encourage! Observe how she responds to your encouragement, and keep doing what works for her. If something changes, and she's no longer responding to the same thing she used to, you may need to do some work to figure out what's behind it.

Observing also means watching, quite literally. If you've been open and honest with your daughter throughout this process, she should be quite used to you being in the bathroom while she's busy, and vice versa. You should be comfortable with her being around while you're doing your thing.

Observe her while she's busy and make sure she's still doing things the right way and doesn't need extra help. If she seems like she needs a bit more work, don't make her feel bad for what she's doing, though. Gently guide her in the right direction. At the same time, allow her to keep observing you if she needs to. Act natural while in the bathroom, but don't sneak in behind her to watch, though! Just be normal, wash your hands, look in the cupboard, or have a conversation.

If you notice any hint of discomfort, it's always a good idea to chat to your daughter and ask her if she's okay or if there's anything she's unhappy about. She may not be able to explain the details, but she could be able to tell you if anything is making her uncomfortable or if she's worrying about things.

Dealing With Accidents

It can be tempting to assume that your little girl is an expert at this potty thing now and you no longer need to think about it.

But remember, you've just taught her the basics over this weekend. She now knows when and where she needs to go, but getting her timing right is going to take a bit of work.

Remember, bladder and bowel control isn't fully developed until around the age of 4, so if your little girl is younger, this could be the reason accidents happen. Young children understand when they need to go, and where they need to go, but the timing from feeling it to getting to the toilet is where things might fall apart a little.

Accidents don't mean that you've failed, or that your child doesn't learn, or that the 3-day method is useless! Not at all. As you go forward from the potty-training weekend, your child's body and brain have a bit of adjusting to do. They've just learned this new process, but as they go forward, there may be times when signals get crossed.

A common reason for accidents in the first few weeks is that your child gets a feeling that they need to potty while they're on the playground or immersed in a game or with a toy. They're having such fun they don't really want to stop, so they ignore the urge. Before they know it, they can't hold it anymore and whoops….out it comes.

Another common occurrence is being in public. Shy children are especially prone to these accidents. When there are other people around, whether you're in the shopping mall or at a friend's house, they may just be too shy to tell you they need to go.

Or it could just be that she's not paying attention and has forgotten for the moment that she's not wearing a diaper, releasing it before she remembers.

Whatever the reason is behind your little one's accident, you're one step closer to it being the last accident!

The 3-day method is a foundation. It teaches your daughter to start paying attention to her body and understanding how to feel when she needs to go. But it's not a rock-solid habit. Just like any new skill, it needs constant work going forward, and there will be slip-ups.

In reality, the learning curve is just beginning when your child sets foot out of the house on that first day after the 3-day weekend. She may have done brilliantly over the weekend, but remember she was learning in a controlled environment with only a few potential outcomes. Now, she's in the real world where the potty is further away and other people are all around. That's a little different, and not as easy!

When accidents happen, it could be instinct to yell, get upset, or even punish your daughter. I urge you to fight these feelings! Remain positive, kind, and calm, and treat your little one with love.

To be honest, I believe it's even more important to be patient in the weeks following than it was over the actual weekend. If you react in a negative way now, your daughter may start to feel anxiety that she's not good enough. This could lead to a regression, so it's in everyone's best interests to keep it loving as you go through these weeks.

If accidents are frequent or tend to happen in public, you can put a little more effort into getting your daughter comfy with different types and styles of toilets. The fear of an unknown toilet could be one of the reasons she's having accidents.

Many moms I know carry an entire home in their baby bags, so it shouldn't be a big deal to take your toilet seat potty attachment with you when you're out and about. Of course, you can't carry it in your purse, but you can keep it in the car for when you visit friends or family members. This is also an effective method if your child is great with the potty, but not so comfy with the toilet seat attachment.

Try feeding your child a high-fiber snack and a juice box before leaving home. This will start the process going, and then it's just waiting until they need to go. Remind them gently to let you know if they need to go. When they tug on your sleeve, simply

78

take them to the toilet, place the seat in position, and let them do their thing.

Once they've done this a few times in a public toilet (because the only other option was to have an accident), they may be more comfortable using the big toilet at home, and in turn, getting more comfortable when they're out.

Another common reason for your child not wanting to go in the big toilet is that they're scared of the height when they sit on it. Their potty is low to the ground and nonthreatening, but the big toilet could be quite intimidating. You will need to find a way to combat this and reassure your daughter that it's perfectly safe.

Also, most toddlers won't be able to go a full night without an accident, at least for a few months after the weekend. You could let her sleep in a diaper, and help her get excited about dressing in her big-girl panties in the mornings, until the accidents stop completely.

You'll need to keep in mind that every child will move along this path differently, and at a different pace. It's important to be attentive and observe, observe, observe! If you can pick up where your daughter has weaknesses, you can shift your after-the-weekend training to work directly on those things. You can even do a few 3-day potty-training exercises to reinforce her learning and comfort level.

Remember, however things go moving forward, your child is doing better than they were before the weekend! You need to be there to guide her along the way until she can confidently and capably do this thing on her own.

What to Do in the Case of an Accident

- **Be Prepared**

Always expect an accident. That may sound negative, but that's certainly not how I mean it! But in order to best deal with accidents, it's super important to be prepared. That way, you won't be shocked and horrified when it does happen, and you'll be quite ready to clean up and move forward.

If your child doesn't have an accident, then it's all happiness and celebrations! To be safe, keep a change of clothing, some cleaning supplies like tissues or wet wipes and sanitizer spray, and some bags to carry dirty clothes in.

- **Stay Calm**

As mentioned before, whatever you do, try your hardest to not draw attention to your child or yourself. If she's had an accident, she will most likely be feeling ashamed and like she's done something wrong. Drawing any more attention to her will only worsen the situation.

Do everything you can to stay calm, and get her cleaned up as quietly as possible. Remember, staying calm is not just about what you say! Keep a demeanor of calm too. Your child can feel your frostiness if you're annoyed and/or just remaining silent. A quiet word of encouragement is always a good thing.

- **Don't Punish Your Child**

You'll understand as you've read through this book that I'm an advocate of treating our children with love and patience and only giving positive reinforcement. Punishing your child can be damaging to their self esteem, and could actually have very negative consequences.

Parents, I know how it feels to have put days of hard work into this and then have to deal with your child having an accident. Depending on how your mood is on the day, it can be tempting to give your child a spank or admonish them.

Please, resist! I can guarantee you have more chance of undoing all the good you've done by displaying anger or impatience. Treating your child with love and patience in this situation will make all the difference to her confidence.

She'll go forward knowing that she hasn't disappointed the parents she loves. She'll figure this out, knowing that she has loving and supportive parents by her side.

Regression

It can happen that a child who has been effectively potty-trained loses their way and needs to wear a diaper again because they can't get it right. This isn't common, though, and please don't assume this is happening if your child has an accident or a few!

A few accidents doesn't mean your daughter needs to start wearing a diaper again. It may seem incredibly frustrating and feel like she will never pass that hurdle, but trust in the process.

In serious cases, though, a child could completely forget everything they've learned or develop a sudden fear of going to the toilet or potty. If she's having an accident every single time she has to go and there are no successful potties, that's somewhat more concerning.

The good news is that there's always a reason behind a regression. If you can figure out what that is, the chances of fixing it are high. Unfortunately, it can sometimes be difficult to figure out what exactly is behind it.

Parents, if your daughter regresses, I know it can be a huge blow. It can feel like you've failed her, or done something wrong in the whole process. Even worse, you could suddenly worry that you've done something to dash her self-esteem and wreck this whole process!

But don't worry. The weekend training certainly hasn't gone to waste. Remember, this is just foundational work. If your daughter showed progress, it means the foundations have stuck in her mind. Although a regression may cause her to "forget" how to properly go potty for a while, she hasn't truly forgotten.

The foundations are still there, and when she has dealt with whatever has caused the regression, she can go right back to standing on those foundations.

What I can tell you is that, although it feels like all your hard work has been for nothing, this process of regressing is infinitely harder on your child than it will be on you. Don't fall into the trap of assuming she's being lazy or stubborn! Of course, some kids are just like that. But if that's not your child, there's no reason she should suddenly develop a stubborn streak that only manifests itself when she needs to potty!

Your daughter is probably feeling anxiety. She may even be feeling ashamed and not good enough. You've spent a whole weekend teaching her, and been offering constant positive reinforcement, and she's just not getting it right. Don't think that she's not smart enough to understand how important this is and what impact it may have. Toddlers are much smarter than we give them credit for, and they also pick up quite easily on their parents' feelings.

If your daughter has suddenly stopped progressing and you feel this is a regression and not just a string of accidents, here's what to do.

What to Do

- **Stay Calm**

When a regression happens, you'll most likely feel disappointed, defeated and incredibly frustrated. I want you to know that it's completely normal to feel these things! The key is not to display these feelings to your daughter.

When she's not around, you can rage and cry all you need to. But when you're with her, clamp any negative emotions or reactions down. Go out of your way to stay calm and loving.

Remember, calm doesn't necessarily mean quiet. You can remain quiet, but if there's a black cloud of anger over your head, your daughter is going to feel terribly bad.

Stay calm with your words and actions, but do your best to stay calm in feeling too. Remind yourself that this is not the end of the world. Every child gets potty-trained in the end - even if they've had a regression.

- **Don't Punish Your Child**

When you've seen good results before, it can be very tempting to assume that your daughter is just being stubborn and punishing her may snap her out of it. But children don't generally make an effort to be lazy.

Also, do you think your child really wants to be dealing with a wet, dirty, smelly diaper on multiple occasions just to trick you into diapering them up again, so they can be lazy about pottying? No! A dirty diaper is uncomfortable, as are the feelings that come with it and the looks from other people. Toddlers are not above feeling ashamed.

Don't add punishment to the already tense situation. I can guarantee that your child's feelings are already enough punishment for them. Be loving.

- **Stick to Positive Reinforcement**

I don't mean praising your child for not getting it right. Positive reinforcement can be tough to get right when your child is doing something they shouldn't be, whether by choice or not.

You obviously can't praise your daughter for regressing. But as always, you shouldn't be negative about it either. Which leaves the middle ground - neutrality.

This should mean no praising, but also no punishment. This is a quiet support on the side while your child goes through this.

I'd like to stress that you shouldn't encourage your child by saying that they've done it before, so they can do it again. This could possibly make them feel worse about not being able to do it now!

Simply stay by their side, support quietly, and…

- **Ask Your Child Why It Happened**

Regression isn't just something that happens for no reason. Don't let that scare you, though. While there can be big and scary reasons behind it, there can also be small and seemingly insignificant reasons that are obviously much bigger to your little one than they seem to you.

While most parents may immediately assume that something huge is wrong, something as small as another child at daycare laughing at something that may or may not have been your child's toilet habits could set off a regression.

If your daughter can talk to you about this, ask her to tell you why she can't go potty anymore.

Understand that whatever has caused your little girl to stop progressing is a trauma in her mind. It may not necessarily be a physical trauma. But it means that something has caused (and may still be causing) your child enough anxiety that she can't do what she used to be able to do anymore.

If she tells you, that's great! You can start working towards fixing it. If she can't tell you, that's okay too. Simply wait and support her in every way you can. Wait until she can either tell you, or she's comfortable enough to begin re-training.

- **Sympathize With Your Child**

You don't need to tell her that you know how she's feeling or be too verbal about knowing how she feels. Just let her know that it's okay. Be sympathetic but not pandering.

She'll want to know that she's not a failure, that she's not broken. She'll need to know that you still love her the same and aren't completely disappointed. You'll need to make sure she knows these things!

- **Start Training Again**

When you're certain that she is feeling comfortable and less anxious, you can begin training again. You'll most likely need to start at the beginning again. You can set up another full weekend if you felt it went well last time. You may need to tweak it slightly, so she doesn't recognize the trick and instantly feel not good-enough again.

Take your time, though. Don't expect miracles. You'll need to be even gentler and more caring than the first time round.

Her body already knows what to do. It's just a case of making her feel comfortable enough to do it naturally again.

- **If Necessary, Take Her to the Pediatrician**

If you can't find any good reason for the regression, and if you're seeing no light of day with introducing re-training, it may be worth a trip to the doctor. A quick check-up could reveal potential medical reasons that may be playing a part.

Common Problems (and Their Solutions)

Whether you're learning to play an instrument, learning to drive, or learning how to poop in the right place, there will be challenges encountered along the way. These are to be expected! If your child learns quickly and moves forward with little to no problems, you can consider yourself a lucky parent indeed!

Most problems are quite harmless and can be fixed fairly easily. Often, the biggest problem is the frustration that comes with them! Parents can begin to feel like they're doing the wrong thing, teaching the wrong methods, or just have a defective child (yes... we're all guilty of feeling these things sometimes).

But rest assured, in most cases neither you nor your daughter are doing anything wrong. If you've been following the steps in this book, you're most likely on exactly the right track. Your child is most likely also just a little more curious than most, and you'll need to put in some extra work to overcome these minor speed bumps.

Here are some problems you may come across and how to fix them quickly.

Your Daughter Doesn't Recognize When She Needs to Go

I know. You may be wondering how hard it can possibly be, considering we all know how uncomfortable it can be to have that pressure that's impossible to ignore! But it often happens that children begin to recognize when they need to poop, but can't yet feel when they need to pee. This is perfectly normal and nothing to worry about!

It can be a little frustrating, but it will right itself along the way. Pooping often comes with gassiness, pain, and discomfort. These things are quite a bit easier to be aware of than the subtle twinge of a full bladder!

It's actually very common for children to learn to recognize and control their bowels months before they learn to do the same with their bladder. If your daughter isn't quite recognizing when she needs to pee, she's quite normal!

You'll need patience for this. There's really nothing you can do but wait until it sorts itself out. Don't assume that she's doing something wrong or missing the point! At this point, her brain and body are getting to know each other, and it could take some time to figure things out.

When the bladder is full, it sends an electrical signal to the brain telling it that it needs to be emptied. The brain gets this message and realizes that it needs to display this physically. Once it's decided what to do, it sends a signal back to the body which causes that full-bladder discomfort.

When you're an adult and your brain and body have been communicating for decades, this exchange happens naturally and at the speed of light. But children don't quite have it down yet. Between their developing brains and bodies, one of those electrical signals could go a little wrong and be misinterpreted or missed altogether.

Bowel movements are quite a bit more noticeable than peeing. It makes sense then that the urge to poop would be easier for your little girl to feel than the subtle hint to pee.

This is another thing you'll need to wait out. You can't hurry the brain-body connection!

She Resists Going to the Bathroom

What we're talking about here is not resistance to the potty-training process. This is resisting going potty because the toy/game/situation is exciting, and she simply doesn't want to miss out on anything by going to the bathroom!

This can result in frequent accidents. In these cases, the only problem you need to be concerned about is distraction.

It's important to know that there's a big difference between resistance to being potty-trained and simply getting distracted and resisting putting down what she's busy with to go to the toilet!

If your daughter is very active, this is something to watch out for. She may be doing really well learning to listen to her body and act when the urge comes, but if she's immersed in an activity that she's excited about she could be so interested that she forgets to pay attention to the subtle feelings. By then, it's too late!

After a few accidents happen this way, she will begin to realize why it's happening. Her body-brain will begin to adjust for it. As she develops she'll also be able to hold it in for longer, which will make this problem much easier to deal with.

She's Afraid of the Toilet

Toilets are weird things. They're strangely shaped and make a heck of a noise when you push that lever or button. Is it any wonder children can have a fear of them?

What usually happens in your child's mind is the fear of being sucked into the bowl when it flushes, especially if they've seen the water whirling away. Perhaps this is a primal fear to avoid us getting stuck in sinking sand, but it's a real worry for very young children.

Remember, kiddies are not only much smaller than we are, but their imaginations are wildly more active than ours. When we hear the toilet flush, we think nothing of it. When a toddler hears this thing whoosh, their brain kicks into gear and perceives a threat. Maybe a tidal wave, maybe a dinosaur. Either way, the noise is scary and that churning water means they could get slurped down there easily.

Help make your daughter more comfortable with the flushing of the toilet by letting her flush it while you're sitting on it. This will help her to understand that it doesn't eat humans, and that it's perfectly safe for mom, so why shouldn't it be safe for her?

If you want her to be able to see how it works, let her flush a piece of toilet paper down and watch it flow away, explaining to her that this is what happens to her pee or poop.

She Tries to Touch Her Pee or Poop

This is a simple case of curiosity! Their poop is usually in their diaper, and they don't see it. Seeing it in the potty may involve some kind of fascination. It's not disgusting or creepy. It's just your child doing what comes naturally to them - learning.

However, it is important to stop this kind of behavior early on. Simply explain to them that they shouldn't play with it. When she's still learning, you should be remaining in the bathroom until the pee or poop is flushed away completely. This will give you the opportunity to notice any poop-play and get a handle on it immediately.

It may not be easy to persuade her to leave it alone. Toddlers can be quite insistent, and if she's a stubborn one, telling her she can't play with it will only make her want it more!

If this is a problem, I advise making a big deal of disposing of the poop so your daughter can see that you're actively trying **not** to touch it.

Exaggerating your facial expressions and body language can do wonders. Pick up the potty and look at what's inside, then look away quickly and exaggerate your facial expression. Pretend to sniff it and make an even more horrified face!

Empty the poop into the toilet, taking extra care not to touch it and again, exaggerate what you're doing. If you need to remove it, emphasize every movement you make. Make sure that she watches you and sees **you** making an effort not to touch it.

If you see her making a move to touch it, gently take her hand and make a "yucky" face. Do this gently but firmly. It's meant to be a light but firm gesture to show that you're protecting her from something nasty.

Keep doing this, and soon she'll get bored with it. Hopefully, the smell should put her off!

She'll Only Go to the Toilet With One Particular Person

You may find that your daughter is so used to going to the toilet with mom that she refuses to go if you aren't with her. This problem can pop up especially at daycare or if she spends time at a friend or another family member's home. When mom or dad suddenly aren't around, she may panic and try to hold it in, which can lead to accidents and feelings of shame.

If this is a problem your daughter is having, you need to start withdrawing yourself from her potty time, slowly but surely. Begin by leading your child to the toilet as usual, but waiting outside while she does her business. This way, she'll know that you're right there, but she'll also start to build up confidence that she can go by herself.

Let her know that any adult family member or friend can take her to the door of the toilet. If she doesn't want them inside with her, she can tell them to wait outside. It's a good idea to work on this with a friend or family member that your child is familiar with but doesn't trust quite as much as they do you.

Don't forget to tell your daughter never to go to the toilet with a stranger, though!

Conclusion

You've come to the end of this blueprint, and I hope that you're reading this conclusion knowing that potty-training is far less complicated and scary than it seemed when you began this book!

You should now know that there's a way to do it effectively and efficiently, with as little stress and anxiety as possible, and in a way that's both fun for your child and loving. And in just a weekend!

If you're still a little on the fence about whether or not the 3-day method works, you don't have to take my word for it! Here are some word-for-word reviews from real parents the world over who have had success teaching their children this method (*3 Day Potty-Training Review » Potty-Training a Stubborn Child*, n.d.):

- "I potty-trained my daughter last week, and she's still doing great. My daughter will be 3 this coming Monday and she's a bit hard headed so I wasn't sure if this would really work for her. I took the day off of work on Friday to start and it was pretty hard, as you said it would be. By Saturday afternoon I couldn't see how I wasn't going to be able to use Pull-ups for her at daycare. However, Sunday came and she didn't have a single accident all day. I told my daycare provider what I had done and all she needed to do to help. I think she was a bit skeptical herself. It's now Friday, 5 days in daycare, and she hasn't had a single accident. My daycare lady was so impressed."
  - Jennifer
- "I am a stay at home mom and have just potty-trained Lindsey using your method. Lindsey is a 3 years and 9 month little girl who is wonderful in every way…but, is

VERY stubborn and definitely has a mind of her own. She is a very quirky child - she wants to do what she wants to do and is on her own agenda. A trait that will serve her well later in life (she'll probably be one of our great leaders), but it definitely does make parenting her a challenge. We started this WONDERFUL program last Wednesday and have been accident free since Saturday!! All weekend she has been going on her own or telling us in her own way that she has to go." - Michelle

- "The old saying of "seeing is believing" absolutely applies to us. Our little Emilee is so headstrong we thought no way is this program going to work. The first day she had about 8 accidents. My wife was ready for the accidents and it did not seem that Emilee was ever going to understand using the potty. On the second day we made some headway. She still had about 5 accidents but seemed to start to understand by telling us when she needed to go potty. On the third day I was blown away when Emilee told us to stay where we were because she wanted to use the potty by herself. I will never forget what happened next. A little voice called to us from the bathroom saying, "Guys." We all responded to her call saying "Yeah?" and then that little voice came back and said "I went potty." Joyful cheers rang from the living room and songs of praise fell from heaven. On the fourth day she had one accident involving poop. My wife changed her and used your instructions as far as what to say to her and from that point on she now does that on the potty. She has had two accidents since that day and both happen usually when she is sleeping or just waking up. What I like about these two accidents is how it really bothers her and last night she woke up in the middle of the night around 1am and told my wife she had to go potty and she did. We now have more freedom and can't wait for our 6 month old to reach that age of potty-training." - Tim and Diana

There you go! It's a fact - the 3-day method really works! (for stubborn children as well as more easygoing ones). By simply setting aside three days of your time and placing all your focus on your daughter, you're teaching her exactly how to listen to her own body. Taking this time is a huge step closer to helping your daughter become a fully independent little human!

The most important thing about this method is that it affords your child the freedom to come to realizations about their own body without constant pushing and forcing from their parents. It's as natural a process as we can make it to teach them how to do it. All you need to do is be there to help your child understand what's happening and how to deal with it. Once she understands that she can't just pee or poop in her pants, it's as simple as flipping that switch in her brain that tells her when and where she needs to go.

There's no anxiety, no humiliation, no annoyance. Just a weekend filled with happiness and time spent with mom and dad, plenty of yummy snacks, games, and at the end of the weekend, a new skill learned.

So, moms and dads, are you ready to put in three days of effort and put dirty diapers behind you? If you answered no…well, I have no words! I have a suspicion you may have said yes, though, and there's good news - you have this blueprint and these tools right here at your fingertips. All that remains is for you to take action and put them to good use.

When your child has overcome this milestone, I'd love to hear about it! Please leave a review on Amazon if this book has helped make the process easier, and let me know how well your little girl is doing.

Best of luck and remember - do it all with love!

References

3 Day Potty-Training Review » potty-training a stubborn child. (n.d.). 3 Day Potty-Training. http://www.3daypottytraining.com/w/t/potty-training-a-stuborn-child/

Bureau of Labor. (2020). *EMPLOYMENT CHARACTERISTICS OF FAMILIES -2019.* https://www.bls.gov/news.release/pdf/famee.pdf

Choby, B. A., & George, S. (2008). Toilet Training. *American Family Physician, 78*(9), 1059–1064. https://www.aafp.org/afp/2008/1101/p1059.html#:~:text=Spock

Dewar, G. (2010). *The science of toilet training: What research tells us about timing.* www.parentingscience.com. https://www.parentingscience.com/science-of-toilet-training.html

Meltzoff, A. N. (1999). *Born to Learn: What Infants Learn from Watching Us.* http://ilabs.washington.edu/meltzoff/pdf/99Meltzoff_BornToLearn.pdf

National Center for Biotechnology Information. (2019). Potty-training: Overview. In *www.ncbi.nlm.nih.gov.* Institute for Quality and Efficiency in Health Care (IQWiG). https://www.ncbi.nlm.nih.gov/books/NBK279296/#:~:text=Research%20suggests%20that%20it%20could

Souders, B. (2019, July 4). *Parenting Children with Positive Reinforcement (Examples + Charts).* www.positivepsychology.com. https://positivepsychology.com/parenting-positive-reinforcement/

CPSIA information can be obtained
at www.ICGtesting.com
Printed in the USA
LVHW100828120323
741430LV00002B/246

9 781953 631121